DIET IN HEALTH AND DISEASE

DIET IN HEALTH
◇ AND DISEASE ◇

RATIONALE AND PRACTICE

By

RUTH STRATHEARN DICKIE, M.S., R.D.
Associate Professor and Director of Continuing Education
Dietary Services
University of Wisconsin Center for Health Sciences

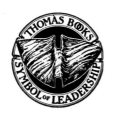

CHARLES C THOMAS • PUBLISHER
Springfield • Illinois • U.S.A.

Published and Distributed Throughout the World by

CHARLES C THOMAS ● PUBLISHER

BANNERSTONE HOUSE

301-327 East Lawrence Avenue, Springfield, Illinois, U.S.A.

© *1974, by* RUTH DICKIE

ISBN 0-398-02899-0 (Cloth)

ISBN 0-398-02919-9 (Paper)

Library of Congress Catalog Card Number: 73-7875

With THOMAS BOOKS careful attention is given to all details of manufacturing and design. It is the Publisher's desire to present books that are satisfactory as to their physical qualities and artistic possibilities and appropriate for their particular use. THOMAS BOOKS will be true to those laws of quality that assure a good name and good will.

Library of Congress Cataloging in Publication Data

Dickie, Ruth S.
  Diet in health and disease: rationale and practice.

  1. Diet in disease. 2. Nutrition. 3. Dietaries. I. Title. [DNLM: 1. Diet. 2. Diet therapy. 3. Hospital food service. 4. Nutrition. WB400 D552d 1973]

RM216.D56   613.2   73-7875

ISBN 0-398-02899-0

ISBN 0-398-02919-9 (pbk.)

Printed in the United States of America

A-1

PREFACE

THIS MANUSCRIPT WAS UNDERTAKEN to meet the requests of dietitians throughout the state who were participating in the Institutional Food and Nutrition Radio-Telephone Conferences sponsored by the Department of Postgraduate Medical Education. As the literature was searched to formulate answers to questions submitted to me as director of the program, I realized the need for a book written for the practitioner. Such a book would have more information on the rationale of nutritional practices than is found in the traditional dietetic manual; it should have greater emphasis of food selection and use than is found in most textbooks.

Many sources were consulted for information on the composition of foods found in the marketplace. The Wisconsin Department of Agriculture, the Wisconsin Alumni Research Foundation, the University of Wisconsin Department of Food and Dairy Science, and Oscar Mayer and Company of Madison all answered many questions and gave freely of their knowledge. Many processors of food and beverage products sold nationally provided laboratory analysis on their products. This assistance was greatly appreciated.

To provide maximum freedom in adapting food plans, the concepts on which current practices are based are reviewed. Diet therapy may involve quite different approaches in practice. Every institution has its own mission and needs. An outpatient facility would give highly individualized nutrition counsel whereas a large hospital food service would be quite routinized. Of necessity, diets for the hospital operation will be more restricted to cover a broader range of similar need. Likewise, practices in a nursing home may be different in many respects from practices in a large referral hospital. The patient with acute symptoms of disease may require quite different treatment than the individual with stabilized chronic symptoms of the same disease process.

Dietary practices are placing much greater emphasis on the

responsibilities of the individual as a participant in the development of his program of long-term nutritional care. Greater consideration is being given to the family and the community as providers of this type of nutritional care. This means greater emphasis on understanding the *why* as well as the *how* of treatment. Communications and cooperation among all health related agencies in the community are vital to success. The dietitian should coordinate the nutritional care component of the total program.

Diet in Health and Disease: Rationale and Practice is written for health professionals concerned with the delivery of nutritional care. References have been selected to acquaint the reader with a broad range of library resources, and in some instances to note the developmental stages of our present concepts. Some of these references are general reviews. Others are for the student who wishes a quick introduction into problems being investigated and authors publishing reports concerning research in each area. Textbooks used by physicians and nutritionists have been listed in the Appendix, with a short notation as to their content or usefulness. Some books have been listed in one section of the text only. Rather than repeat a whole list of references for each section, publications which are used throughout the text (such as Watt and Merrill 1963, Robinson 1972, and Goodhart and Shils 1973) have full biographical citation the first time they appear only. The annotated list of these publications appear in Appendix IV.

Many reference sources are available to individuals pursuing their own continuing education. Most medical libraries will provide a printout of a National Library of Medicine computer based Medical Literature and Retrieval System search ("Medlars" search) on a particular subject. For the practitioner not close to a medical library, many medical schools have an Extension Service which will process requests for a Medlars search, and will loan books and journals. Frequently local institutional or public libraries will handle requests for technical publications on a free Interlibrary Loan basis.

Both the American Hospital Association and the American Dietetic Association maintain a library service for their members. The journal of each association carries a section devoted to recent publications. Every issue of the Journal of the American Dietetic Association carries a whole section of abstracts of articles related to nutrition and food service in a broad range of journals.

A word about the text is in order. The punctuation system adopted by the New England Journal of Medicine has been used: no periods are used in abbreviations and Index Medicus style is used in abbreviation of titles.

The staff (including many disciplines) of the University of Wisconsin Center for Health Sciences have provided consultation on current practices. Some of these individuals were noted as consultants. Many others whose suggestions were just as useful, but were less closely related to any one section, have not been mentioned by name. ES Gordon, M.D. Professor of Medicine, contributed viewpoints on the fat modified diets.

Miss Dorothy Ridler, M.S., Nutrition Consultant of the Wisconsin Department of Health, Retired, deserves special mention for her continuing participation in the preparation of this manuscript. Her broad experience, vision, and editorial review have been invaluable. My sister, Helen Dickie, M.D. also performed a valuable service in bringing to my attention the advances and controversies related to nutrition in medicine. She gave me an increased awareness of research groups from which reports could be expected, and the journals in which such reports were likely to be found. Barbara Johnson Smith and Marilyn Ribbe Swanson have freely shared their specialized knowledge in providing diets for children with phenylketonuria. Annette Gormican, Ph.D. Associate Professor of Nutritional Sciences has provided suggestions and counsel. And Mrs. Jeanne Evert has patiently typed from hard-to-read copy. To all a debt of gratitude is due.

Ruth Strathearn Dickie

TABLES

CONTENTS

DIET IN HEALTH AND DISEASE

SECTION I

GUIDELINES
FOR GOOD NUTRITION

I N 1943 THE FOOD and Nutrition Board of the National Research
Council published the first edition of the recommended daily
dietary allowances designed for the maintenance of good nutrition
of practically all healthy people in the United States. Since then
there have been revisions to keep pace with the findings in the
sciences of nutrition. The most recent edition is the eighth, published in 1973.

These recommendations have been a foundation for planning
food supplies and for guiding their use in the feeding of individuals,
groups, and populations. They are the bases for the food plans in
this publication.

Included in this section are the following:

**THE RECOMMENDED DAILY DIETARY ALLOWANCES, 1973
(SEE TABLE I-1)**

A Daily Food Guide. This is a translation of the dietary allowances into kinds and quantities of foods to be eaten daily given in
terms of four major food groups: The Meat Group, the Milk
Group, the Vegetable-Fruit Group, and the Bread-Cereal Group
(*Food for Fitness,* 1967). These basic food groups, and the groups
of Fats and Sugars are listed in detail.

The Food Exchange System. This offers a tool for quick calculation of nutrient values and permits flexibility in food selection. The
original listings by the American Diabetes Association (1950) are
included in this section with a few additions. Exchange groups of
foods, adapted from this system, are included in appropriate diets.

3

TABLE I-1

FOOD AND NUTRITION BOARD, NATIONAL ACADEMY OF SCIENCES—NATIONAL RESEARCH COUNCIL

RECOMMENDED DAILY DIETARY ALLOWANCES,[1] Revised 1974

Designed for the maintenance of good nutrition of practically all healthy people in the U.S.A.

	(years) From Up to	Weight (kg)	Weight (lbs)	Height (cm)	Height (in)	Energy (kcal)[2]	Protein (g)	Vitamin A Activity (RE)[3]	Vitamin A Activity (IU)	Vitamin D (IU)	Vitamin E Activity[5] (IU)
Infants	0.0-0.5	6	14	60	24	kg x 117	kg x 2.2	420[4]	1,400	400	4
	0.5-1.0	9	20	71	28	kg x 108	kg x 2.0	400	2,000	400	5
Children	1-3	13	28	86	34	1300	23	400	2,000	400	7
	4-6	20	44	110	44	1800	30	500	2,500	400	9
	7-10	30	66	135	54	2400	36	700	3,300	400	10
Males	11-14	44	97	158	63	2800	44	1,000	5,000	400	12
	15-18	61	134	172	69	3000	54	1,000	5,000	400	15
	19-22	67	147	172	69	3000	54	1,000	5,000	400	15
	23-50	70	154	172	69	2700	56	1,000	5,000		15
	51+	70	154	172	69	2400	56	1,000	5,000		15
Females	11-14	44	97	155	62	2400	44	800	4,000	400	12
	15-18	54	119	162	65	2100	48	800	4,000	400	12
	19-22	58	128	162	65	2100	46	800	4,000	400	12
	23-50	58	128	162	65	2000	46	800	4,000		12
	51+	58	128	162	65	1800	46	800	4,000		12
Pregnant						+300	+30	1,000	5,000	400	15
Lactating						+500	+20	1,200	6,000	400	15

[1] The allowances are intended to provide for individual variations among most normal persons as they live in the United States under usual environmental stresses. Diets should be based on a variety of common foods in order to provide other nutrients for which human requirements have been less well defined. See text for more-detailed discussion of allowances and of nutrients not tabulated.

[2] Kilojoules (KJ) = 4.2 x kcal.

[3] Retinol equivalents.

[4] Assumed to be all as retinol in milk during the first six months of life. All subsequent intakes are assumed to be one-half as retinol and one-half as B-carotene when calculated from international units. As retinol equivalents, three-fourths are as retinol and one-fourth as B-carotene.

[5] Total vitamin E activity, estimated to be 80 percent as a-tocopherol and 20 percent other tocopherols. See text for variation in allowances.

Years From up to	Ascorbic Acid (mg)	Folacin[6] (μg)	Niacin[7] (mg)	Riboflavin (mg)	Thiamin (mg)	Vitamin B6 (mg)	Vitamin B12 (μg)	Calcium (mg)	Phosphorus (mg)	Iodine (μg)	Iron (mg)	Magnesium (mg)	Zinc (mg)
Infants													
0 - 0.5	35	50	5	0.4	0.3	0.3	0.3	360	240	35	10	60	3
0.5- 1.0	35	50	8	0.6	0.5	0.4	0.3	540	400	45	15	70	5
Children													
1 - 3	40	100	9	0.8	0.7	0.6	1.0	800	800	60	15	150	10
4 - 6	40	200	12	1.1	0.9	0.9	1.5	800	800	80	10	200	10
7 -10	40	300	16	1.2	1.2	1.2	2.0	800	800	110	10	250	10
Males													
11 -14	45	400	18	1.5	1.4	1.6	3.0	1200	1200	130	18	350	15
15 -18	45	400	20	1.8	1.5	2.0	3.0	1200	1200	150	18	400	15
19 -22	45	400	20	1.8	1.5	2.0	3.0	800	800	140	10	350	15
23 -50	45	400	18	1.6	1.4	2.0	3.0	800	800	130	10	350	15
51+	45	400	16	1.5	1.2	2.0	3.0	800	800	110	10	350	15
Females													
11 -14	45	400	16	1.3	1.2	1.6	3.0	1200	1200	115	18	300	15
15 -18	45	400	14	1.4	1.1	2.0	3.0	1200	1200	115	18	300	15
19 -22	45	400	14	1.4	1.1	2.0	3.0	800	800	100	18	300	15
23 -50	45	400	13	1.2	1.0	2.0	3.0	800	800	100	18	300	15
51+	45	400	12	1.1	1.0	2.0	3.0	800	800	80	10	300	15
Pregnant	60	800	+2	+0.3	+0.3	2.5	4.0	1200	1200	125	18+[8]	450	20
Lactating	80	**600**	+4	+0.5	+0.3	2.5	4.0	1200	1200	150	18	450	25

Water-Soluble Vitamins — *Minerals*

[6] The folacin allowances refer to dietary sources as determined by *Lactobacillus casei* assay. Pure forms of folacin may be effective in doses less than one-fourth of the RDA.

[7] Although allowances are expressed as niacin, it is recognized that on the average 1 mg of niacin is derived from each 60 mg of dietary tryptophan.

[8] This increased requirement cannot be met by ordinary diets; therefore, the use of supplemental iron is recommended.

Courtesy of the National Research Council, National Academy of Sciences.

A DAILY FOOD GUIDE

After making nationwide studies of food consumption the United States Department of Agriculture developed food plans for healthy people based on the recommended dietary allowances of the National Academy of Sciences-National Research Council. In this plan the foods to include daily are divided into four groups. Within each group foods have a general likeness in nutrient value; and each of the four groups is expected to furnish a large part of the daily allowance of one or more key nutrients. Studies made in developing these plans have shown that if the recommended amounts of foods of key nutrient content are included, the recommended allowances for all nutrients are likely to be achieved even though the remainder of the diet may be made up of foods of lower nutrient content (Page and Phipard, 1957).

This dietary plan is not the only way the recommended dietary allowances may be met, but since it is based on the food habits in this country it seems to be the best framework for meals for most people. More than the minimum number of servings from some of the basic food groups will ordinarily be eaten. Other foods, such as fats and sugars, are customarily part of most meals. These other foods are added as desired, or in the case of a diet prescription, as recommended, to complete the day's meals.

This Daily Food Guide is one way to choose food wisely. With it, the essential nutrients may be obtained from a variety of everyday foods.

How To Use This Guide

In using this Daily Food Guide the main part of the day's food is selected from four broad food groups. To this are added other foods as needed to make meals more satisfying and appealing. Some pointers for guidance in using this plan are as follows:

1. Choose at least the minimum number of servings from each of the broad food groups. Serving sizes may differ; small for young children, extra large (or seconds) for very active adults or teenagers. Pregnant and nursing women also require more food from these groups.

2. Make choices within each group according to suggestions given on the following pages. Foods within each group are similar,

but not equal, in food value. On selective menus, force choice of foods which provide key nutrients by listing together two or more foods which are a "good" to "excellent" source of that key nutrient.

3. Choose the additional foods to round out the meals both from foods in the four groups and from foods not listed in these groups. These additional foods should add enough calories to complete the energy needs for the day. Children need enough food energy to support normal growth; adults need enough to maintain body weight at a level most favorable to health and well-being.

4. Try to have some protein-containing food at each meal.

Vegetable-Fruit Group

Foods Included

All vegetables and fruit. This guide emphasizes those that are valuable as sources of vitamin C and vitamin A.

Sources of Vitamin C

Good Sources: Grapefruit, grapefruit juice; orange, orange juice; cantaloup; guava; mango; papaya; raw strawberries; broccoli; brussels sprouts; green pepper, sweet red pepper.

Fair Sources: Honeydew melon; lemon; tangerine; tangerine juice; watermelon; asparagus tips; raw cabbage; collards; garden cress; kale; kohlrabi; mustard greens; potatoes and sweet potatoes cooked in the jacket; spinach; tomatoes; tomato juice; turnip greens.

Sources of Vitamin A (Carotene—provitamin A)

Dark-Green and Deep-Yellow Vegetables and a Few Fruits: Apricots, beet greens, broccoli, cantaloup, carrots, chard, collards, cress, kale, mango, persimmon, pumpkin, spinach, sweet potatoes, turnip greens and other dark-green leaves, winter squash.

Contribution to the Diet

Key nutrients from this group are: vitamins C, A, riboflavin, folic acid, iron, and magnesium.

Amounts Recommended

Four or more servings every day, including:

One serving of a good source of vitamin C or 2 servings of a fair source.

One serving, at least every other day, of a good source of vitamin A. If the food chosen for vitamin C is also a good source for vitamin A, the additional serving of a vitamin A food may be omitted.

The remaining 1 to 3 or more servings may be of any vegetable or fruit, including those that are valuable for vitamin C and vitamin A. If calories are limited, the green leafy vegetables are recommended for the additional servings because they give a high nutrient return for the calories invested. Count as 1 serving: one-half cup of vegetable or fruit, or a portion as ordinarily served, such as 1 medium apple, banana, orange, or potato one-half of a medium grapefruit, one-third of a cantaloup 5 inches in diameter, or the juice of 1 lemon.

One serving of fruit or vegetable from the list of good sources of vitamin C and one serving from the list of sources of vitamin A will provide more than half of the recommended dietary allowance for ascorbic acid, and three-fourths or more of the recommended dietary allowance for vitamin A.

Each serving of food recommended in this section for vitamin A contains a minimum of 2500 IU of vitamin A value in the form of carotene, or half the recommended daily allowance. Some of the foods contain three times this amount. Color is a general guide for this vitamin. The deeper the yellow as in carrots, or the darker the green as in spinach or chard, the greater the quantity of carotene present.

Recent emphasis has been on expressing vitamin A values in terms of retinol equivalents. Rodriguez and Irwin (1972) use the value of 1 IU of vitamin A as equivalent to 0.3 micrograms retinol, and 1 microgram all-trans-carotene as equivalent to 0.167 micrograms all-trans retinol. However, they point out that other mixed carotenoids with vitamin A activity are equivalent to .0835 micrograms all-trans retinol. The 1973 *Recommended Dietary Allowances* list both international units and retinol equivalents.

FAO/WHO Technical Report Series no 41 (1967) reviews factors in the consumption pattern which influence the availability and utilization of vitamin A in foods. Little data are available on the influence of stress or disease on utilization.

Milk Group

Foods Included

Milk, fluid whole, skim, evaporated, buttermilk; dry.
Cheeses, all kinds, natural or processed.
Ice cream. Ice milk.

Contribution to the Diet

Key nutrients from this group: calcium, magnesium, riboflavin, protein, vitamin A, vitamin B_{12}, and vitamin D if milk is fortified.

Amounts Recommended

Some milk every day for everyone. Recommended amounts are given below in terms of fluid whole milk:

	8-ounce cups
Children under 9	2 to 3
Children 9 to 12	3 or more
Teenagers	4 or more
Adults	2 or more
Pregnant women	3 or more
Nursing mothers	4 or more

Two cups of milk provide for the adult approximately:

2/3 of the recommended dietary allowance for calcium.
1/4 of the recommended dietary allowance for protein.
1/2 of the recommended dietary allowance for riboflavin.
1/5 to 1/4 of the recommended dietary allowance for magnesium.

Without milk, the diet will not meet the recommended dietary allowance for calcium and will probably be low in riboflavin and tryptophan.

A sizable portion of the vitamin A recommended daily is expected to come from whole milk. Because vitamin A is soluble in fat the removal of cream (and hence vitamin A) makes it advisable when using skim milk to use that fortified with vitamin A.

Adult requirements for vitamin D have not been determined. Casual exposure to sunlight probably meets the low adult needs, and attention should be given only to those who work at night or who are not exposed directly to sunlight.

Milk fortified in vitamin D and skim milk fortified in both vitamins A and D are recommended for general use so that those members of the family who need vitamin D will have it. Buttermilk and chocolate drink are not usually fortified. Dry milk powder is not always fortified with vitamins A and D. Dry skim milk is an excellent low-cost food and may be used extensively, but if the dry milk is not fortified with vitamins A and D other plans should be made to secure these important nutrients.

Meat Group

Foods Included

Beef; veal; lamb; pork; variety meats, such as liver, heart, kidney; sausages; poultry; fish and shellfish; eggs.

As alternates: dry beans, dry peas, lentils, nuts, peanuts, peanut butter.

Contribution to Diet

Foods in this group are valued for their protein, iron, thiamin, riboflavin, B_6, B_{12}, and niacin. Legumes are rich in magnesium, but low in methionine and vitamin B_{12}.

Five ounces of foods from the Meat Group provide approximately:

3/4 of the recommended dietary allowance for protein.
1/2 of the recommended dietary allowance for iron for men; 30 percent for women 15-50 years old.
1/3 of the recommended dietary allowance for B_6.
3/4 of the recommended dietary allowance for B_{12}. (Based on all meat)

Protein provides the required amino acids. Supplement legumes with milk or egg.

For best and most economical utilization of the eight amino acids essential for adults, all eight should be present at each meal. This explains the recommendation that a food from the milk or meat group that contains protein of high biological value should be included in all three meals. Thiamin is widely distributed in foods, and no one food group is its chief provider. Pork is one of the richest sources, and in its lean forms, may be used to advantage in restricted diets. Riboflavin is provided in meat and eggs, and also in foods from the three other basic food groups. One 3-ounce serving of meat provides approximately half as much riboflavin as one cup of milk. Niacin is present in significant quantities in meat. Also, meat and milk contain tryptophan, a precursor of niacin, and are therefore doubly important in providing this vitamin. Cheese and/or milk, if used in sufficient quantity in a meal and in addition to the recommended daily amount from the Milk Group, may be considered an alternate for the protein provided by meat.

Amounts Recommended

Two or more servings every day.

Count as a serving: 2 to 3 ounces of lean cooked meat, poultry, or fish, all without bone; 2 eggs; 1 cup cooked dry beans, dry peas, or lentils; 4 tablespoons peanut butter.

Bread-Cereal Group

Foods Included

All breads and cereals that are whole grain, enriched, or restored; check labels to be sure.

Contribution to Diet

Foods in this group furnish worthwhile amounts of protein, iron, thiamin, riboflavin, niacin, vitamin E, and food energy.

Amounts Recommended

Four servings or more daily. Or, if no cereals are chosen, include an extra serving of bread or baked goods. This will make five servings from this group daily. Count as a serving: 1 slice of bread; 1 ounce ready-to-eat cereal; 1/2 to 3/4 cup cooked cereal such as cornmeal, grits, macaroni, noodles, rice, spaghetti.

The Bread-Cereal group, if whole grain or enriched, is important because of its broad nutritional contribution at low cost rather than any outstanding contribution of one or a few nutrients. These foods contain some protein and may be used as a valuable source of this nutrient in low cost diets. Cereals should always be accompanied by a food from the milk or meat group for good utilization of amino acids.

Three slices of whole wheat bread and 1 serving of rolled oats will contribute approximately the following to the recommended dietary allowances:

1/5 to 1/4 of the protein for the adult man or woman.

1/4 of the iron for the adult man, and 1/8 of the iron for the adult woman except over 50 years of age.

Other Foods

Everyone will use some foods not specified in the basic food groups. These foods include fats such as butter, margarine, salad and cooking oils; sugars such as cane, beet, maple syrup, honey, and corn syrup; and unenriched grain products. They are often ingredients in baked goods and food combinations. Fats, oils, and sugar may be added to foods during preparation or at the table. These other foods supply calories, and certain ones contribute to the total nutrients of the day's foods.

Fats and Oils

Margarine	Oils, cooking or salad
Butter	Salad dressings made with oil
Lard	Salt pork
Mayonnaise	Vegetable fats and shortenings

Butter contains vitamin A in seasonal variation; margarine according to the year-round average of butter. Butter and margarine may be used interchangeably in the diets except those that are restricted in saturated fats (modified fat, low cholesterol diets). Margarines made chiefly with vegetable oils are used in these diets because of their higher ratio of polyunsaturated fats to saturated fats (PUFA/S).

Vegetable oils (other than coconut) are exceptional sources of vitamin E. It is wise to include some vegetable oil among the fats used. Margarines provide vitamin E in amounts depending on the oils used in them and in the method of manufacture.

Fats and oils are composed of fatty acids. Vegetable oils contain linoleic fatty acid which is an essential nutrient.

Sugars and Sweets

Honey	Sorghum
Molasses	Jellies, jams, preserves
Syrups; corn, maple, etc.	Candies
Sugars of all kinds	Confections made with cereals and candy

These foods are concentrated carbohydrates; they provide calories and little else of nutritive value. Honey, molasses, and the fruit products—jellies, jams, preserves—contain small amounts (traces only in some) of minerals and/or vitamins. They serve a purpose as sweetening agents when combined with other foods as in custards, puddings, cookies.

Combined Foods

These are combinations of foods prepared together to be served as a single menu item. They include entrees such as baked chicken with noodles, hearty salads such as chef's salad, and desserts such as apple pie. Ingredients for these dishes may include foods from the major food groups, and would then contribute to the day's recommendations for these foods. Other ingredients in these food combinations may be refined cereals, and/or fats and/or sugars.

Entrees such as casseroles in the hospital menus were planned

TABLE I-2

CALORIE AND PROTEIN VALUES OF AVERAGE SERVINGS OF
SOME COMBINED FOODS

	Approximate Amount	Approximate Weight Ounces	Calories Per Serving	Protein Per Serving Grams
Entrées				
Beef and vegetable stew*	2/3 cup	5 to 6	270	27
Beef and rice, baked*	2/3 cup	5 to 6	290	20
Chicken and noodles*	2/3 cup	5 to 6	300	19
Macaroni and cheese	2/3 cup	5 to 6	287	11
Desserts				
Angel food cake*	1/12 of 8" diameter cake	1-1/3	110	3
Apple pie	1/7 of 9" diameter pie	4-1/2	350	3
Cooky, sugar*	3" diameter	1	106	1
Cupcake, chocolate icing	2-1/2" diameter	1-1/4	130	2
Custard, baked*	1/3 cup	3	95	4
Date bar*	2" x 2" x 1-1/2"	2-1/2	300	2
Gelatin dessert	1/2 cup	4	70	2
Ice cream*	1 dixie cup	2 (3 fluid)	112	2
Ice milk, hardened	1/3 cup	2	67	2
Lemon sponge*	1/2 cup	3	280	5
Peach crisp*	1/2 cup	4	400	2
Pumpkin pie	1/7 of 9" diameter pie	4-1/2	275	5
Sherbet*	1/3 cup	2-2/3	101	1
Vanilla pudding*	1/3 cup	3	105	5

*Calculated from recipes.

to provide, per serving, two ounces of cooked meat, fish, or egg or the equivalent amount of protein from the Milk Group; this in addition to the recommended daily amount from the Milk Group.

Caloric values for average servings range from about 100 to 400 for the food combinations for which nutrient estimates were made. Some of these (marked with an *) are included in Table I-2. For these the food values of Watt and Merrill (1963) and the recipes in use at the University Hospitals were used. Values for the others are from USDA's *Nutritive Value of Foods,* Home and Garden Bulletin 72, 1970.

Iodine

Iodine is an essential nutrient for all people. Since it has been leached from the soil in some areas of the United States products grown in these areas may be deficient in iodine.

Iodized salt is a safe and effective way of providing iodine. The cost of iodized and non-iodized salt is the same, and containers are usually placed side by side in the grocery stores. Purchasers should be cautioned to check the labels.

Fluids

At least 7 to 8 cups of water or other fluids daily for adults. The National Research Council (1973) recommends one milliliter water per calorie of food for adults, 1.5 ml per calorie of food for infants as a reasonable allowance under ordinary circumstances. *Special attention to water needs must be given to infants on high protein formulas; to comatose patients; to those with fever, polyuria, or diarrhea, or who are consuming high protein diets; and to all persons in hot environments.*

THE FOOD EXCHANGE SYSTEM AND FOOD EXCHANGE LISTS

The foregoing daily food guide applies to the selection of food for the general population. The objective is the inclusion of foods providing key nutrients in the daily meals of all people.

A food exchange system was developed in 1950 by committees of the American Diabetes Association and the American Dietetic Association in cooperation with the Chronic Disease Program of the

Public Health Service, Department of Health, Education, and Welfare. The objective of this plan was to provide a system of exchanges of food on the basis of protein, fat, carbohydrate, and calorie content. It was originally intended for calculation of diets in diabetes mellitus. In this plan foods are grouped in six lists:

List 1. Milk   List 4. Bread, cereals, starchy vegetables
List 2. Vegetables   List 5. Meat
List 3. Fruit   List 6. Fat

Each food in a list, *in the quantity shown,* is approximately equal to the others in that list in available glucose and may be exchanged for any other in that list. Therefore, the lists have been designated as Exchange Lists, and each food on a list is called a *food exchange.* A few foods markedly lower in fat are noted and additions to equalize are given in terms of fat exchanges.

Quantities of foods are given in easy-to-measure units related to the usual way foods are purchased, prepared, and served. Average values for calories and for protein, fat, or carbohydrate are given for a serving in each of the six lists. Robinson (1972, page 690.) gives rounded weights in grams of the exchanges.

Since 1950 the use of the food exchange system has been extended to include meal planning for diets other than for diabetes and for quick calculations of food intakes in respect to protein, fat, carbohydrate, and calories. The overall nutritional values of the foods in each list vary so that correlation of these lists with the recommendations of the daily food guide is important in making diet plans. The publication *Meal Planning with Exchange Lists (1956)* includes the six lists, methods of measuring, and some recipes.

Recent publications (Gormican 1971, Revell 1971) give exchanges for many new items. Many food processors have calculated glucose equivalent food exchanges for their products and will provide them on request.

A list of lean meat items for use in planning diets restricted in fat is presented in this section following the six standard exchange lists.

List 1. Milk Exchanges

One exchange of milk contains 12 grams carbohydrate, 8 grams protein, 10 grams fat, and 170 calories. One cup equals 8 fluid ounces.

Type of Milk	Amount	Add to Day's Food
Whole milk, plain or homogenized	1 cup	
Skim milk	1 cup	2 fat exchanges
Evaporated milk, undiluted	1/2 cup	
Powdered whole milk	1/4 cup	
Powdered skim milk (non-fat dry milk)	1/4 cup	2 fat exchanges
Buttermilk, made from whole milk	1 cup	
Buttermilk, made from skim milk	1 cup	2 fat exchanges
Yogurt, plain, made with whole milk	1 cup	
Yogurt, plain, made with low fat milk	1 cup	1 fat exchange

Skim milk, partially skimmed milk, and buttermilk made with skimmed milk have the same food values as whole milk except that they contain less fat and fat soluble vitamins. See additional fat exchanges to be included in the day's food if one cup of skim milk, or buttermilk, or yogurt made with low fat milk is used.

Vegetable Exchanges

The vegetables have been divided into three groups according to their approximate yield in available glucose:

List 2A. These contain little carbohydrate, protein, or calories. In the amount usually eaten their contribution in the foregoing nutrients is considered negligible, but they are important for minerals and vitamins.

List 2B. These contain 7 grams carbohydrate, 2 grams protein, and 35 calories per serving.

The third group, potatoes, parsnips, and other starchy vegetables, are included in the list of Bread-Cereal Exchanges (List 4) since they have values in protein and carbohydrate similar to bread.

List 2A Vegetables

When eaten raw the quantities of these vegetables (except tomatoes) are not limited. Restrict tomatoes to one medium-size tomato or 1/2 cup tomato juice at a meal. If List 2A vegetables are cooked, 1 cup may be used at a time without counting calorie values; or 2 cups may be considered an exchange for 1 serving of a List 2B vegetable.

Asparagus	Greens:	Lettuce
Broccoli*	Beet greens*	Mushrooms
Brussels sprouts	Chard*	Okra
Cabbage	Chicory greens*	Peppers*
Cauliflower	Collards*	Radishes
Celery	Dandelion greens*	Sauerkraut
Cucumbers	Kale*	String beans, young
Eggplant	Mustard greens*	Summer squash
Escarole	Spinach*	Tomatoes
French endive	Turnip greens*	Watercress*

*Good sources of vitamin A, present as carotene.

List 2B Vegetables

One-half cup equals one exchange; 7 grams carbohydrate, 2 grams protein, 35 calories. One-half cup can be substituted for 1/2 Bread-Cereal Exchange.

Beets	Pumpkin*
Carrots*	Rutabagas
Onions	Squash, winter*
Peas, green	Turnips

*Good sources of vitamin A, present as carotene.

List 3. Fruit Exchanges

One exchange of fruit contains 10 grams carbohydrate and 40 calories. These servings are for fruit that is fresh, dried, cooked, canned, or frozen but with no sugar added. Look at the label on the can or package to be sure that it says *unsweetened* or *no sugar added*.

	Amount
Apple (2″ diameter)	1 small
Applesauce	1/2 cup
Apricots, fresh	2 medium
Apricots, dried	4 halves

	Amount
Banana	1/2 small
Blackberries	1 cup
Raspberries	1 cup
Strawberries*	1 cup
Blueberries	2/3 cup
Cantaloup* (6″ diameter)	1/4
Cherries	10 large
Dates	2
Figs, fresh	2 large
Figs, dried	1 small
Grapefruit*	1/2 small
Grapefruit juice*	1/2 cup
Grapes	12
Grape juice	1/4 cup
Honeydew melon, medium	1/8
Mango*	1/2 small
Orange*	1 small
Orange juice*	1/2 cup
Papaya*	1/3 medium
Peach	1 medium
Pear	1 small
Pineapple, raw, diced	1/2 cup
Pineapple juice	1/3 cup
Plums	2 medium
Prunes, dried	2 medium
Raisins	2 tablespoons
Tangerine*	1 large
Watermelon, diced	1 cup

*Good sources of vitamin C: 30 mg/100 gm or over.

List 4. Bread-Cereal-Starchy Vegetable Exchanges

(Generally referred to as "bread exchange"
or "bread-cereal exchange.")

One exchange contains 15 grams carbohydrate, 2 grams protein and 70 calories. This list includes breads, cereals, crackers; dried beans and peas, and some higher carbohydrate vegetables and other foods. Small servings of sponge cake and ice cream are also included. Other dessert type foods can be added on a glucose equivalent basis if the composition is known. Each one of the following servings counts as 1 bread-cereal exchange.

	Amount
Bread or similar product	
Bagel, 2 oz each	1/2 bagel
Biscuit, baking powder, plain	
2″ diameter, 1 oz	1
Bread: white, wholewheat or rye	1 slice
Cornbread or similar	1-1/2″ cube or 1-1/2 oz
Muffin, 2″ diameter, 1-1/3 oz	1
Pancake, 6″ diameter, 1-1/2 oz	1 cake
Popover, about 2 oz	1
Roll, soft or hard, plain	1/2 or 25 gm
Waffle, 7 inch diameter	1/2 or 40 gm
Cereals (The following are approximately 20 gm dry weight)	
Cereals, cooked	1/2 cup
Dry, flake, and puff types	3/4 cup
Rice, corn grits, cooked	1/2 cup
Spaghetti, noodles, macaroni, etc. cooked	
	1/2 cup
Cornstarch	2 tbsp or 16 gm
Crackers	
Graham, 2-1/2″ square	2 or 20 gm
Matzos, 6-1/4 x 6-1/2″	2/3 piece or 20 gm
Oyster	1/2 cup or 20 gm
Saltines, 2″ square	5 or 20 gm
Soda, 2-1/2″ square	3 or 20 gm
Round, thin, 1-1/2″	6 or 20 gm
Rye, whole grain, 1-7/8 x 3-1/2″	3
Pretzel	2/3 oz
Flour	3 tbsp or 20 gm
Sugar (4 gm per tsp)	3-1/2 tsp or 15 gm
Vegetables, dried	
Beans, peas, dried, cooked	1/2 cup
(includes lima, navy, split peas, cowpeas, etc)	

	Amount
Baked beans, no pork	1/4 cup
Popcorn, popped, plain (6 gm per cup)	3 cups or 1/2 oz
Vegetables, starchy	
Corn	1/3 cup
Parsnips	2/3 cup
Potatoes, white, boiled or baked	1 small
Potatoes, white, mashed	1/2 cup
Potatoes, french fried	1-1/2 oz (8 pieces, 2 x 1/2 x 1/2")
Potato chips, 2" (omit 2 fat exch)	1 oz (15 chips)
Potatoes, sweet, or yams	1/4 cup
Cake sponge, plain,1-1/2" cube	25 gm
Cake, angel, commercial, plain, 1-1/2" cube	25 gm
Doughnut, cake type or yeast (omit 1 fat exch)	1 oz (no sugar coating)
Ice cream (omit 2 fat exch)	1/2 cup or 65 gm
Ice milk (omit 1 fat exch)	
Hardened	1/2 cup or 60 gm
Soft serve	1/3 cup or 60 gm
Sherbet	1/4 cup or 50 gm

Other fruits and vegetables can be used in place of bread-cereal exchanges.

2B vegetable list—1/2 cup = 1/2 bread-cereal exchange
1 cup = 1 bread-cereal exchange
Fruits, list 3 —1-1/2 exchanges (portions as listed) = 1 bread-cereal exchange

Measure the vegetables on the Bread-Cereal-Starchy Vegetable Exchange list after they have been cooked. Whole grain, enriched, or fortified breads and cereals are good sources of iron and the B vitamins.

List 5. Meat Exchanges

One meat exchange contains 7 grams protein, 5 grams fat, and 75 calories. Each one of the following servings counts as one meat exchange. If any food is added, such as fat or flour in preparation of the food, it is taken from the day's allowance in that food group. These quantities refer to ready-to-eat weights. Bones and extra fat are not counted in the serving weight. The selection of items is not limited and does not reflect any regional preference.

	Amount		*Amount*
Meat & poultry, cooked	1 ounce	Fish, fresh or frozen,	
Beef, lamb, pork, ham,		cooked	1 ounce
veal, fowl, liver, etc.		Cod, haddock, halibut,	
		pike, perch, flounder,	
		sole, etc.	
Cold cuts, 4½″ x 1/8″	1 ounce	Salmon, tuna, crab,	
Salami, liverwurst,		lobster	1/4 cup
bologna, minced ham,		Shrimp, clams, oysters	5 small
luncheon loaf		Sardines	1 ounce
Frankfurter, 8 to 9/lb	1	Cheese, cheddar type	1 ounce
Egg, 8 per lb	1	Cottage cheese	1/4 cup
		Peanut butter	2 tbsp

This list represents a variety of foods within a range of protein and fat content. The frequency of use (weighting) of items at the high or low end of the range will increase or decrease the protein and fat averages of the group.

Most fish are lower in protein and fat than most meats. If used often the amount of an exchange may be adjusted accordingly. For cooked fish (plain) 1½ ounces is roughly equivalent in protein and fat to 1 ounce of cooked meat.

Cold cuts and cooked sausages are lower in protein and higher in fat than the exchange value shown above. To reflect these differences, if used often, 1½ ounces of any item of this type may be used as 1 meat exchange, *but* 1½ fat exchanges must be taken from the day's fat allowance.

About 4 or 5 ounces of most raw meats, under average conditions of shrinkage, will provide 3 ounces of cooked meat. See USDA Home Economics Research Report No. 37 (1969) for a guide to calculating amounts to buy to provide a given weight of cooked meat.

List 6. Fat Exchanges

One fat exchange contains 5 grams fat and 45 calories. Each of the following servings counts as one fat exchange. Teaspoon and tablespoon are standard size. All measurements are level.

	Amount		Amount
Bacon, cooked crisp (18-20 slices to a pound raw)	2 slices, 15 gm	Cream cheese	1 tablespoon
		French dressing	1 tablespoon
Butter or margarine	1 teaspoon	Mayonnaise	1 teaspoon
Cream, light	2 tablespoons	Oil, cooking fat	1 teaspoon
Cream, heavy, whipping	1 tablespoon	Nuts	6 small
		Olives	5 small
Cream, heavy, whipped	2 tablespoons	Avocado, 4″ diameter	1/8th

Note: One pound raw bacon will yield 0.31 pound cooked, ready-to-serve bacon (Oscar Mayer Products Nutritional Data, Oscar Mayer and Co., Madison, Wis. 1972).

LEAN MEAT EXCHANGE LIST

The following Lean Meat Exchange List is designed for use when the fat in the diet is restricted. This list is patterned after the exchange lists developed by the American Diabetes Association, the American Dietetic Association, and the U.S. Dept. of Health, Education, and Welfare.

In this Lean Meat Exchange List the selection of meat, fish, and poultry is limited to lean items. They are to be trimmed of fat before cooking and at the table, and cooked without added fat (unless taken from diet allowance). Skin of poultry or fish is excluded; and an egg is not included as an exchange in this list. The protein and fat of one ounce each of some representative foods were averaged and the resulting values rounded to 8 grams protein and 3 grams fat. (See *Protein, Fats, and Cholesterol in a Selected Group of Meats, Poultry and Fish*, Table VI-13 in Section VI for calculation of these values.)

The National Institutes of Health in their dietary management of hyperlipoproteinemia (Fredrickson et al., 1971) uses the values of

8 grams protein and 3 grams fat per ounce of cooked product when a choice of lean meats, fish, and poultry is allowed. When pork, beef, and lamb are restricted to three 3-ounce servings in a week, the value of one ounce cooked product of this selection (which includes veal, chicken, other lean items) is listed as 8 grams protein and 2 grams fat.

Lean Meat Exchange List

One exchange of any of the following foods is counted as 8 grams protein, 3 grams fat, and 60 calories.

Under average conditions of shrinkage and waste 4 to 5 ounces of raw, boneless, lean meat will provide about 3 ounces of cooked meat.

	Quantity for exchange
Meat, lean cuts only without bone, cooked:	1 ounce
Beef, lamb, fresh or cured pork, veal	
Chicken or turkey, no skin	
Fish, fresh or frozen, cooked:	1 ounce
Salmon, canned	1 ounce
Tuna, cnd in water, solids & liquids	1 ounce
cnd in oil, drained solids	1 ounce
Shellfish:	
Crabmeat, canned or cooked	1½ ounces
Clams, drained solids	1½ ounces
Lobster, canned or cooked	1½ ounces
Scallops, steamed	1½ ounces
Shrimp, frozen or dry pack or drained solids	1½ ounces
Oysters, raw, drained	3 ounces
Cheeses:	
Cottage, creamed, uncreamed, low fat	1/4 cup
Cheddar; leave out one fat exchange	1 ounce
Parmesan; 5½ tablespoons	2/3 ounce
Swiss; leave out 1 fat exchange	1 ounce

SOURCES OF NUTRIENTS IN U. S. FOOD SUPPLY

Statistics compiled from the U. S. Department of Agriculture surveys of food consumption in the United States (see Table I-3) provide information useful in food planning. Most noteworthy is the fact that milk, meat, grain, and the vegetable-fruit groups each make a significant nutrient contribution to the diet. The protein, mineral and vitamin contribution of each in relation to the money invested, or the food energy (calories) provided, is quite different for each group. In this respect they complement each other toward meeting the total nutrient needs.

Where therapeutic restrictions, gross food dislikes, or food customs severely restrict items from one or more of the basic four food groups, well formulated plans must be made to furnish from other sources an equivalent portion of nutrients eliminated. If limitations are severe, mineral and/or vitamin supplementation may be required. Ways are shown for adapting food selection and food preparation to meet various therapeutic needs. Further changes in meal patterns may be essential to meet the individual's need or preferences.

A comparison of the nutrient contribution from each food group with the relative expense shows that milk products and grain (cereal) foods give particularly good nutritional returns per dollar spent. These are also the food groups where there is a broad price range for items within the group, allowing adjustment to family economic levels. In the milk group, savings can be made by purchasing dry milk and the less expensive cheeses. If non-fat dry milk is purchased, a product fortified with vitamins A and D should be selected.

Within the grain group, the less refined products, particularly the whole grain cereals which require cooking, generally are the cheaper. At the lower economic levels, grain products supply a higher proportion of the family's nutrient needs. Products enriched with B vitamins and iron are a wise selection. The table shows that in 1970 grain products contributed 18 percent of the protein in the American diet, 27 percent of the iron, 34 percent of the thiamin, 14 percent of the riboflavin and 23 percent of the niacin. The latest (1965) available data showed an expenditure of only 12 percent of the food dollar for this food group.

The yield of edible meat from different cuts varies widely, influenced by type (steak, roast, etc.), grade, and cutting practices in specific markets. Foods from the meat group give a good nutritional return even though they take the largest portion of the food dollar.

TABLE 1-3—CONTRIBUTION OF MAJOR FOOD GROUPS TO NUTRIENT SUPPLIES AVAILABLE FOR CIVILIAN CONSUMPTION, 1970
(Preliminary data)

Food Group	Food Energy Pct.	Protein Pct.	Fat Pct.	Carbohydrate Pct.	Calcium Pct.	Phosphorus Pct.	Iron Pct.	Magnesium Pct.	Vitamin A Value Pct.	Thiamin Pct.	Riboflavin Pct.	Niacin Pct.	Vitamin B6 Pct.	Vitamin B12 Pct.	Ascorbic Acid Pct.
Meat (including pork fat cuts), poultry, and fish	20.3	41.5	34.9	.1	3.6	26.2	30.8	13.7	23.3	29.5	25.5	47.1	47.1	70.1	1.1
Eggs	2.2	5.8	3.3	.1	2.6	6.0	6.0	1.4	6.8	2.5	5.9	.1	2.2	9.3	0
Dairy products, excluding butter	11.3	22.1	12.7	6.9	75.8	36.0	2.3	21.8	11.3	9.7	42.4	1.6	9.4	20.6	4.5
Fats and oils, including butter	17.7	.1	42.3	[2]	.4	.2	0	.4	8.4	0	0	0	.1	0	0
Citrus fruits	.8	.4	.1	1.7	.8	.6	.8	1.9	1.3	2.5	.5	.8	1.1	0	24.5
Other fruits	2.4	.6	.3	5.1	1.3	1.2	3.7	4.0	6.6	2.0	1.6	1.9	5.8	0	12.0
Potatoes and sweetpotatoes	2.8	2.4	.1	5.5	1.0	4.0	4.6	7.3	5.7	6.6	1.8	7.4	12.0	0	20.3
Dark green and deep yellow vegetables	.2	.4	[2]	.5	1.5	.6	1.6	2.0	20.8	.9	1.0	.6	1.7	0	8.4
Other vegetables, including tomatoes	2.4	3.2	.4	4.5	4.8	4.8	9.2	10.2	15.3	7.0	4.5	5.9	9.2	0	29.2
Dry beans and peas, nuts, soya flour	2.9	5.0	3.5	2.1	2.7	5.7	6.4	10.9	[2]	5.6	1.8	6.8	4.2	0	[2]
Flour and cereal products	19.8	18.1	1.4	35.8	3.4	12.6	26.6	18.1	.4	33.7	14.3	22.5	7.0	0	0
Sugars and other sweeteners	16.6	[2]	0	37.1	1.1	.2	5.6	.4	0	[2]	[2]	[2]	.1	0	[2]
Coffee and cocoa[3]	.7	.4	1.2	.6	1.0	1.8	2.6	7.8	[2]	.1	.7	5.2	.1	0	0
Total[4]	100.0	100.0	100.0	100.0	100.0	100.0	100.0	100.0	100.0	100.0	100.0	100.0	100.0	100.0	100.0

[1] Percentages were derived from nutrient data which include quantities of iron, thiamin, and riboflavin added to flour and cereal products; quantities of vitamin A value added to margarine and milk of all types; quantities of ascorbic acid added to fruit juices and drinks. [2] Less than 0.05 percent. [3] Chocolate liquor equivalent of cocoa beans. [4] Components may not add to total due to rounding.

From Friend, B: Nutritional Review. National Food Situation, NFS-134, USDA, Washington, DC, Nov. 1970.

Knowledgeable buying practices can materially increase the nutrient return from each dollar spent on meat, poultry or fish. Legumes are an economic alternate, but should be supplemented with additional milk.

Good nutrition counsel can help families establish lifetime purchasing and eating habits which contribute to their health and well being. Accurate knowledge is particularly important to individuals under economic or metabolic stress. Food plans are outlined in this manual to assist individuals in adapting their therapeutic diets to family food plans.

REFERENCES

References used in compiling this text are included in the following manner:

1. References specific to a given subject, and cited references, are listed at the end of the section to which they apply.

2. General references are included in the appendix, some with annotations.

Some of the general references were used throughout the manual, especially those with the rationale of dietary practice, with recommended dietary allowances, and with calculations of nutrient estimates. To avoid repetition these are listed once under the heading of General References in Appendix IV.

The student is referred to bibliographies given in the listed publications for background information, and to medical indexes for more recent articles by investigators.

REFERENCES

Agri Research Serv: *Food for Fitness: A Daily Food Guide*, revised. Washington, DC, USDA Leaflet No 424, 1967.
—————: *Family Food Buying: A Guide for Calculating Amounts to Buy and for Comparing Costs.* HERR No 37, Washington, DC, USDA, 1969.
American Diabetes Association, American Dietetic Association, and Chronic Disease Program, Pub Health Serv, Dept of HEW: *Meal Planning with Exchange Lists.* Chicago, Am Diet Assoc; or New York, Am Diabetes Assoc, 1950.
Caso, EK; Stare, FJ: Simplified method for calculating diabetic diets. *JAMA, 133*:169, 1947.

Caso, EK; Stare, FJ: Simplified method for calculating diabetic diets. betic Diet Calculations, American Dietetic Association. Prepared cooperatively with the Committee on Education, American Diabetes Association, and the Diabetes Branch, US Pub Health Serv. *J Am Diet Assoc, 26*:575, 1950.

Dawson, EH; Gilpin, GL; Fulton, LH: *Family Food Buying: A Guide for Calculating Amounts to Buy and Comparing Costs.* HERR No 37. ARS-USDA, 1969.

FAO/WHO: Requirements of vitamin A, thiamine, riboflavin, and niacin. FAO Nutr Meet Report Series No 41, WHO Tech Report Series No 362, Geneva, Switzerland, 1967.

Fredrickson, DS, et al: *Dietary Management of Hyperlipoproteinemia: A Handbook for Physicians,* Rev. National Heart Lung Institute, National Institutes of Health, Bethesda, Maryland, 1971.

Leverton, RS; Odell, GV: *The Nutritive Value of Cooked Meats.* Misc Pub 49. Okla Agri Exp Sta, Okla State Univ, 1958.

Robinson, CH: *Normal and Therapeutic Nutrition,* 14th ed. New York, Macmillan, 1972.

Rodriguez, MS; Irwin, MI: A conspectus of research on vitamin A requirements of man. *J Nutr, 102*:909, 1972.

Watt, BK; Merrill, AL: *Composition of Foods: Raw, Processed, Prepared.* Washington, DC, ARS-USDA, 1963.

GENERAL DIET
AS SERVED IN A HOSPITAL

THE GENERAL DIET OUTLINE given to a patient on discharge from the hospital is designed to meet the needs of a person who is well, not under stress, and who has achieved a desirable body weight. This outline is based on the daily food plan for good nutrition, and adjusted to the appropriate calorie level by the addition of supplementary servings from the major food groups and of suitable amounts of fats and sugars. Since hospitalized patients are under stress this general diet is used in planning hospital menus that have increased amounts of protein and other nutrients.

The hospital general diet is used, wherever practicable, as the starting point for planning diets to meet different age and condition requirements and to make therapeutic modifications. Additions to this diet, subtractions, and food alternates bring this plan within the requirements of most dietary prescriptions.

Daily Plan for Hospital General Diet

Milk Group

Two cups milk. One-third cup half and half, if desired.

Meat Group

Meat, fish, poultry, eggs, and alternates, dry beans and peas, nuts, peanut butter. Five to six ounces divided among the meals. Usual pattern is three ounces (cooked weight) at one meal, two ounces at another, and one ounce or an egg at breakfast.

Vegetable-Fruit Group

Five to six servings, including: one vitamin C food daily, one

28

dark-green or deep yellow vegetable every other day, three to four additional servings. These may be any *other* fruit or vegetable, and need not be different kinds at a meal, or different ones for each meal. Vitamin C and A foods may be repeated in the day.

Bread-Cereal Group

Four servings, whole grain, enriched, or fortified. Usual pattern is a slice of bread at each meal and a serving of cereal at breakfast or combined with other foods at noon or night.

Fats and Oils

Three pats of butter in the day, each one-fifth ounce. One table-spoon salad dressing or less. This is usually a vegetable oil dressing for a salad.

Sugar

One teaspoon sugar (one packet) was included in the calculations.

* * * * * * *

Combined Foods

Four servings in three days. These are entrees, soups, or desserts. (See Combined Foods, Section One). Ingredients may include foods from the milk, the meat, the vegetable-fruit, and the bread-cereal groups; if so they are counted toward the day's total. Additional ingredients may be fats, sugars, refined cereals, flour. One or more of the desserts may be omitted, or a fruit substituted for a reduction of calories.

* * * * * * *

One or more of the desserts may be omitted, or a fruit substituted for a reduction in calories.

The approximate size of the servings is given in the Method of Calculating the Nutrient Estimates in Appendix II. Larger or smaller servings were provided according to the desires, age, or condition of the individual.

The calculated nutrient estimate for calories is 2265 with a distribution of 15% protein, 38% fat, and 47% carbohyrate. (See Table II-1)

Diet in Health and Disease

TABLE II-1
CALCULATED NUTRIENT ESTIMATES OF GENERAL DIETS AS SERVED IN A HOSPITAL

| | | Recommended Dietary Allowances | | |
| | | For 23 to 50 | For 23 to 50 | Hospital |
Nutrients	Unit	Year Man	Year Woman	General Diet
Food energy	Calorie	2,700	2,000	2,265
Protein	gm	56	46	86
Fat	gm	—	—	96
Carbohydrate	gm	—	—	265
Calcium	gm	0.8	0.8	1.1
Phosphorus	gm	0.8	0.8	1.5
Iron	mg	10.0	18.0	14.0
Magnesium	mg	350.0	300.0	301.0
Sodium	mg	—	—	3,952
Sodium mEq				172
Potassium	mg	—	—	2,995
Potassium mEq				77
Vitamin A	IU	5,000	4,000	6,250
Vitamin E		15 IU	12 IU	7.1 mg
Ascorbic acid	mg	45	45.0	80.0
Folacin	mg	0.4	0.4	—
Niacin equivalent	mg	18.0	13.0	14.0
Riboflavin	mg	1.6	1.2	2.1
Thiamin	mg	1.4	1.0	1.5
Vitamin B_6	mg	2.0	2.0	1.8
Vitamin B_{12}	mcg	3.0	3.0	5.0

Vitamin E recommendations by the National Research Council are given in international units; the nutrient estimates for E in the hospital diets were calculated in milligrams since the table used (Ames, 1968) listed milligrams of alpha-tocopheral in 100 grams of a food.

No calculations for the folic acid content of the hospital diets were made. The 1974 recommended dietary allowances are included in the listing of nutrients, and comments on the folic acid content of foods are in Appendix I.

The iron content of the hospital general diet as outlined meets the recommended allowances for men and women over 50 years, but does not meet those for boys 12 to 18 years and for women from 10 to 50 years. Day-by-day selection of foods may not do so.

In order to meet the NRC recommendations, special attention must be paid to iron-rich foods. A diet outline which illustrates this fact follows. The iron value, 12.0 mg, is calculated from H & G

Bul No 72 (1970) and Watt and Merrill (1963). The values shown in this diet outline are the iron content of single items or the average representing a group of common foods. See Average Iron Content of Portions of Foods following.

Diet Plan Showing Average Iron Values

Food or Food Group	Amount	Iron, milligrams
Milk, whole, skim, partly skimmed, buttermilk	2 cups	0.2
Meat, cooked lean muscle tissue	5 ounces	5.0
Egg (3 a week)	3/7 large	0.5
Vegetable, deep green	1/2 cup	1.4
Potato	1 small	0.6
Other vegetables	1/2 cup	0.5
Fruit, fresh, frozen, canned	2 servings	1.0
Bread: white enriched	2 slices	1.2
Whole-wheat	2 slices	1.6
Butter or margarine	As chosen	0
Sugar, granulated	As chosen	0

In summary of the iron content of foods for diet selection:
1. Beef, veal, and pork muscle tissue are good sources of iron but lower than liver, liver sausage, kidney, and heart which have high iron values. Lamb and chicken are fair sources of iron.
2. Legumes and nuts have good iron values. Peanut butter makes a good contribution when one considers frequent use.
3. Dark green vegetables offer a wide selection and good values in iron.
4. Dried fruits have good iron values, and prune juice is especially high.
5. Whole-grain, enriched, or fortified breads and cereals are good sources of iron. Macaroni, noodles, and spaghetti are available with enrichment in iron to the minimum level set by the Food and Drug Administration. Several food processors are fortifying ready-to-eat breakfast cereals to the level of 10 mg iron per ounce. This information is given on the label.
6. Among the sugars and syrups, molasses and sorghum have outstanding iron values and may be used in a variety of ways.

Variability in the Utilization of Food Iron

According to Turner (1970), "the absorption of iron is a complex process." It is influenced by the amount of available iron in the food, its chemical form, and the presence in the diet of other materials which influence absorbability.

Also, there are widespread differences in absorption of iron by individuals. Among the factors influencing absorption are the level of body stores, the condition of the intestinal mucosa, and alterations in digestive secretions. Ascorbic acid plays important roles in facilitating iron uptake in the intestinal tract and in body cells.

Pyridoxine

Brown (1972) recommends that all women using oral contraceptives receive supplemental pyridoxine.

Average Iron Content of Portions of Foods

These values for the iron content of foods represent unweighted averages of items as listed in H & G Bul 72 (1970) and Watt and Merrill (1963). Items seldom used in hospital menus were not included. A less varied selection may yield higher or lower values depending on the choice.

Newer methods of iron assay are being investigated in a number of laboratories. From some early reports (Gormican, 1970) it appears that the iron content of some foods, notably meats, is lower than data listed here. These averages are presented only to provide a general indication of the comparative iron values of foods and to emphasize the care in selection which must be exercised if National Research Council recommendations are to be met. At low calorie levels pharmaceutical supplementation may be necessary.

Foods Ready to be Eaten	*Amount*	*Iron, mg*
Milk Group		
Milk; whole, skim, partially skimmed, buttermilk	1 cup	0.1
Cheese; cheddar, swiss	1 ounce	0.3
Cheese, cottage, not creamed	1/4 cup	0.2
Meat Group: cooked meat, fish, poultry, eggs		
Beef or chicken liver	1 ounce	2.5
Beef heart; fresh or smoked liver sausage	1 ounce	1.6

Foods Ready to be Eaten	Amount	Iron, mg
Pork liver	1 ounce	8.2
Beef, cured or fresh pork, veal; muscle tissue	1 ounce	1.0
Chicken, lamb, sausage products, fish shellfish, turkey	1 ounce	0.5
Eggs	1 large	1.1

NOTE: Meat group quantities are listed in terms of one exchange.

Legumes and Nuts

Cooked dry beans, split peas, lentils; canned or frozen peas, immature lima beans	1/2 cup	2.1
Almonds, cashews, peanuts, walnuts	1 ounce	0.9
Peanut butter	1 Tbsp	0.3

Vegetables, cooked unless otherwise noted

Dark green vegetables	1/2 cup	1.4
Potatoes, white	1 small	0.6
Potatoes, sweet	1 small	0.8
Lettuce, raw crisphead, shredded	1 cup	0.3
Vegetables other than above	1/2 cup	0.5

Fruit

Fresh, frozen, or canned fruit	1/2 cup	0.5
Dried fruit, weight before cooking	2 ounces	2.1
Fruit juices, exclusive of prune juice	1/2 cup	0.4
Prune juice	1/2 cup	5.3
Fruit "drink"	1/2 cup	0.1

Bread-Cereal Group

Bread, white enriched	1 slice	0.6
Bread, white unenriched	1 slice	0.2
Bread, whole-wheat	1 slice	0.8
Bread, 1/3 rye, 2/3 wheat	1 slice	0.4
Cereals, whole-grain or enriched, cooked: cornmeal or grits, farina, oatmeal, rice, rolled wheat	1/2 cup	0.6
Unenriched cornmeal, grits, farina, rice	1/2 cup	0.2
Cereals, ready-to-eat, whole-grain or enriched	1 ounce	1.0

Foods Ready to be Eaten	Amount	Iron, mg
Cereals high in iron by		
special fortification	1 ounce	10.0
Pastas: enriched macaroni, noodles,		
spaghetti, cooked	1 cup	1.3
Fats and Oils		
Butter, margarine, cooking and salad oils	—	0
Sugars, Syrups, Sweetened Foods		
Honey	1 Tbsp	0.1
Jams and preserves	1 Tbsp	0.2
Jellies	1 Tbsp	0.3
Molasses, light, 1st extraction	1 Tbsp	0.9
Molasses, medium, 2nd extraction	1 Tbsp	1.2
Sorghum	1 Tbsp	2.6
Sugar, white	1 Tbsp	Trace
Sugar, brown	1 Tbsp	0.47
Table syrups, light and dark	1 Tbsp	0.8
Gingerbread, 1/9 of 8″ square cake	2 1/3 ounces	1.0
Gingersnaps or molasses cooky	1 ounce	0.6
Oatmeal raisin cooky	1 ounce	0.8

GENERAL DIET DURING PREGNANCY

Concern over the relatively high neonatal and infant mortality rates in the United States compared to the rates in other countries in the western world prompted the National Research Council through a committee on maternal nutrition to study the problem and develop practical recommendations. From epidemiological studies as well as animal experimentation it was found that routine caloric and salt restriction during pregnancy may not be beneficial; in fact, it may have a deleterious effect. High risk groups among expectant mothers were identified and specific plans were made to meet their special nutrient needs.

Recommendations of the Committee on Maternal Nutrition and the Course of Pregnancy (NAS-NRC, 1970; Shank, 1970) are these:

1. An average total weight gain of at least 24 pounds is expected. Weight reduction during pregnancy is undesirable. Weight gain should be watched closely. A sudden sharp rise after the 20th week

of pregnancy may be a sign of water retention and the possible
onset of pre-eclampsia.

2. Severe caloric restriction, because it is inevitably accompanied
by restriction of other nutrients, is potentially harmful to the mother
and the developing fetus. It may impair the neurological development of the infant.

3. Special attention should be directed to providing appropriate
nutrition counsel to these expectant mothers:

    a. The young girl whose own growth is incomplete.

    b. Women who enter pregnancy in a poor state of nutrition.

    c. Those who have poor dietary habits.

    d. Those who are of low socio-economic status.

    e. Those who have been on slimming regimens.

4. Restriction of salt and prescription of diuretics should be
undertaken only after careful consideration.

5. Routine mineral and vitamin supplementation except for iron
and folic acid is of questionable value. Iron supplementation, 30
to 60 mg per day, is recommended during the second and third
trimesters. All pregnant women should have a daily supplement of
0.2 to 0.4 mg folate.

6. The use of iodized salt is recommended in areas where the
soil and water are deficient in iodine.

Indications For Use

The diet outlined is for the second and third trimesters of pregnancy if no dietary restrictions are indicated.

Daily Plan of General Diet During Pregnancy
as Served in a Hospital

Milk Group

Four cups of fortified whole or skim milk. Small additional
amounts from the Milk Group are provided in occasional servings
of milk soups, cheese.

Meat Group

Meat, fish, poultry, eggs, and alternates, dry beans and peas,
nuts, peanut butter. Six to 7 ounces, divided among the meals. The
usual pattern is 3 to 4 ounces (cooked weight) at one meal, 2 to 3
ounces at a second meal, and 1 to 2 ounces at a third.

Vegetable-Fruit Group

Six to 7 servings, including 2 servings vitamin C foods daily, 1 dark-green or deep-yellow vegetable daily, 3 to 4 other vegetables or fruit.

Bread-Cereal Group

Four servings whole-grain, enriched or fortified. Usual pattern is 1 slice of bread at each meal; 1 serving of cereal at breakfast or combined with other foods at noon or night. Occasionally other grain foods such as rice, noodles, crackers, are added or substituted.

Fats and Oils

Two to 3 pats of butter in the day. One-third to 1/2 tablespoon salad dressing made with a vegetable oil.

Sugar

One teaspoon sugar (1 packet) was included in the calculations. Jelly, honey, syrup, may be substituted.

Combined Foods

Four servings in 3 days. These are entrées or desserts (see Combined Foods, Section One). Ingredients may include foods from the foregoing dietary recommendations; if so, they are counted toward the day's total. Other ingredients may be fats, sugars, refined cereals, flour. One or more of the desserts may be omitted, and a fruit substituted, for a reduction in calories.

Note: Iron-rich foods appear on the 3-day hospital menus which were the basis for calculations of nutrient estimates. Without these iron-rich foods the recommended dietary allowance for iron for the pregnant woman may not be met.

In summary, the general diet plan is followed with these additions to meet the increased nutritional needs of the pregnant woman:

1. Two cups milk
2. One serving of a vegetable or fruit that is a good source of ascorbic acid
3. One ounce of meat or alternate

Sodium Restriction

If sodium intake must be restricted during pregnancy, the general plan of the diet for the pregnant woman would be followed but sodium restriction as outlined in the mild sodium restricted diets (2400 to 4500 mg sodium) in Section VI would be used as a guide. See list of products that contain significant amounts of sodium and of foods to avoid in that section. This diet would be prescribed as a mild sodium restricted diet for a pregnant woman.

GENERAL DIET DURING LACTATION

This diet provides for the increased nutritional needs of the lactating woman, and may be used when no dietary restrictions are indicated.

Daily Plan of General Diet During Lactation
as Served in a Hospital

Milk Group

Four cups fortified whole or skim milk. One-third cup half and half, if desired. Small additional amounts from the Milk Group are provided in occasional servings of cheese, milk soups, ice cream.

Meat Group

Meat, fish, poultry, eggs, and alternates, dry beans, dry peas, nuts, peanut butter. Seven to 8 ounces divided among the three meals. Usual pattern is 3 ounces (cooked weight) at each of two meals, and 1 to 2 ounces at a third.

Vegetable-Fruit Group

Six servings, including: 2 servings vitamin C foods daily, 1 serving dark-green or deep-yellow vegetable daily, 2 to 3 other vegetables or fruit.

Bread-Cereal Group

Four servings, whole grain, enriched, or fortified. Usual pattern is 3 slices bread per day and 1 serving of cereal at breakfast or combined with other foods at noon or night. Occasionally other grain foods such as rice, noodles, crackers are added or substituted.

Fats and Oils

Two to 3 pats of butter in the day. One tablespoon salad dressing made with a vegetable oil.

Sugar

One teaspoon sugar (a packet) was included in the calculations.

More than this may be used if desired, or jelly, honey, syrup, substituted.

Combined Foods

Four servings in 3 days, including one high calorie dessert if desired. Ingredients in these combined foods may include meat, vegetables, etc., from the foregoing recommendations. If so, they are counted toward the day's total. Other ingredients may be fats, sugar, refined cereals, flour (see Combined Foods, Section One). One or more of the desserts may be omitted, or a fruit substituted, for a reduction in calories.

TABLE II-2

CALCULATED NUTRIENT ESTIMATES
GENERAL DIETS DURING PREGNANCY AND LACTATION

Nutrients	Unit	Recommended Dietary Allowances		Hospital General Diets	
		Pregnancy	Lactation	Pregnancy	Lactation
Food energy	Calorie	+300	+500	2,641	3,086
Protein	gm	+30	+20	120	134
Fat	gm	—	—	107	142
Carbohydrate	gm	—	—	310	319
Calcium	gm	1.2	1.2	1.7	1.9
Iron	mg	18.0	18.0	20.0	22.0
Magnesium	mg	450.0	450.0	409.0	417.0
Sodium	mg	—	—	4,492	3,956
Sodium mEq				195	172
Potassium	mg	—	—	4,260	4,561
Potassium mEq				109	117
Vitamin A	IU	5,000	6,000	12,475	13,847
Vitamin D*	IU	400	400	400	400
Vitamin E		15 IU	15 IU	8.6 mg	9.0 mg
Ascorbic acid	mg	60.0	80.0	138.0	151
Folacin	mg	0.8	0.6	—	—
Niacin equivalent	mg	+2.0	+4.0	37.0	42.0
Riboflavin	mg	+0.3	+5.0	3.1	4.0
Thiamin	mg	+0.3	+0.3	1.8	1.9
Vitamin B_6	mg	2.5	2.5	2.2	2.3
Vitamin B_{12}	mcg	4.0	4.0	8.0	8.8

*400 IU vitamin D in 4 cups fortified milk.

Note: Without the iron-rich foods included in these menus the recommendation for this mineral for the lactating woman would not be met. The values of common serving portions of some foods that are good sources of iron are listed in the preceding section on the general diet.

In summary, the hospital general diet is followed with the additions listed below to meet the increased nutritional needs of the lactating woman:

1. Two cups of milk

2. One serving of a fruit or vegetable that is a good source of ascorbic acid

3. One serving of a vegetable or fruit that is a good source of vitamin A

4. One serving of meat or alternate

In the three-day hospital menus which were the basis for the nutrient estimates of this diet, one serving each of cantaloup, broccoli, and spinach were included. Each of these contributes appreciable amounts of vitamin A and ascorbic acid to the diet. The inclusion of one of these, or of another food of similar value, will supply the requirement of one serving each of a vitamin A and a vitamin C food.

INFANT FEEDING

Formula Calculation

Infants require at least 1.5 ml fluid per calorie during the first six months of life. This requirement will be met by allowing 2 to 3 ounces fluids per pound of body weight. Requirements are related to the specific gravity of the urine and caloric consumption. As in the adult, water balance of the infant is affected by fluid intake, protein and mineral content of the diet, body temperature, and the metabolic and respiratory control mechanism.

Fevers, vomiting, diarrhea and polyuria are among the many factors which may produce dehydration. Medications may also alter fluid balance.

Fluid for the infant is provided by the milk and water in the formula, foods eaten, and water as such taken between feedings. Most of the child's solid foods will contain 60 to 70 percent water. Many fruits and vegetables will contain 90 percent or more water. Mixed diets will yield about 12 gms water of oxidation per 100 calories (Laupus, 1969, page 127). Cow's milk has a higher protein and mineral content than human milk, so water is generally added to the formula when cow's milk is used. Water is also offered between feedings.

Gastric emptying time for infants will range from 1 to 4 or more hours. Hence frequency of feeding demand differs considerably, generally ranging in intervals of 3 to 5 hours between feedings. Small weak infants may require feedings at shorter intervals.

Quantities of formula taken at one feeding will vary among infants. Laupus (1969) suggests as a general rule adding 3 to the age in months to arrive at the ounces of formula to offer to an infant at one feeding during the first 5 months of life. Robinson (1972, page 312) recommends age in months plus 2. It is not necessary that the baby take all of each formula offered.

The National Research Council recommends 117 calories per kg of body weight for the first 6 months of life, a reduction to 108 calories per kg from 6 to 12 months and a further reduction to 100 calories per kg for 1 to 3 years. The National Research Council's recommendation for protein (2.2 gms/kg from birth to 6 months) is based on use of breast milk. Because of different amino acid composition, larger quantities of protein are required when cow's milk is used. Laupus recommends 1 3/4 to 2 ounces cow's milk per pound of body weight for the first 6 months of life. Robinson (1972, page 312) recommends 1.5 to 2 ounces whole milk. Carbohydrate, usually sucrose or corn syrup, is used to supply the remainder of the caloric requirement in the formula until such time as other foods are added to the diet to provide the necessary calories.

The formula is generally supplemented with vitamin C starting during the second or third week of life, but the time of adding vitamin C and the amount remain at the discretion of the physician. He may recommend using strained orange juice diluted with equal parts of boiled water. Starting from a teaspoon per day, the quantity would then be increased to 3 ounces of orange juice by 3 months.

Vitamin D supplementation also remains at the physician's discretion. It is important that the mother understand that measurements of vitamin supplements must be precise to avoid fat soluble vitamin toxicity.

The Committee on Nutrition of the American Academy of Pediatrics recommends the use of iron-fortified milk formulas and cereals (Lowe et al. 1969). The diet of a normal term infant should provide 10 mg per day of iron at 2 to 6 months to a maximum intake of 15 mg per day at 6 months to a year.

Example of formula calculations for an infant 3 months of age weighing 11 pounds:

1. Fluid requirement for 24 hours (11 x 2 to 3 ounces fluids per pound weight equals 22 to 33 ounces).
2. Whole milk (11 x 1-3/4 to 2 ounces per pound equals 19 to 22 ounces).
3. Fluid requirement (22 to 33 ounces less amount from milk, 19 to 22 ounces, difference is 3 to 11 ounces water to add to formula).
4. Calories recommended (117 per kg equals 585 calories).
5. Other foods will be started as prescribed to meet total caloric need. Some sugar can be added to formula. See *Recent Advances in Therapeutic Diets* (1970), page 123, for a description of proprietary infant formulas.

This formula provides sufficient fluid under ordinary circumstances. In hot environments or under conditions of increased fluid loss, water should be offered between feedings.

Further information on the composition of other milks, various commercial formulas and baby foods, when to add foods to the diet, and serving portions at various age levels will be found in the textbooks cited. The physician will adapt these recommendations to the specific infant. There is considerable variation in the physiological readiness of infants to diet increments.

FOOD FOR INFANTS THREE TO TWELVE MONTHS OF AGE

This diet indicates the foods added to the infant's feedings of milk during the first year of life in order to meet the recommended allowances for nutrients.

Solid food supplements can be started at approximately three months of age. Addition of solid foods to adequate milk diets at an earlier age appears to be of no particular value. At about this age the infant becomes capable of transferring food to the back of the mouth and then swallowing it.

Foods which are good sources of iron and ascorbic acid are added to the diet first since milk is deficient in these factors. If the mother's intake of vitamin C is good (see Diet During Lactation) the breast-fed infant does not require the addition of a fruit juice as a source of ascorbic acid. Also, many prepared formulas contain supplemental vitamin C. Vegetables and fruit which are good sources of minerals and vitamins are the second consideration for food supplementation.

The American Academy of Pediatrics recommends that infants receive 400 international units of vitamin D daily. One quart of vitamin D fortified milk contains 400 IU (or 400 USP units) of the vitamin. Most proprietary infant formulas are similarly fortified.

The National Research Council recommends 35 milligrams ascorbic acid daily during the first year of life. This is generally started in synthetic form in the formula and gradually switched to orange juice. Three ounces of strained orange juice, the kind usually given to infants since it may be taken through a nipple, provides approximately 35 milligrams ascorbic acid. When additional amounts of vitamin D and ascorbic acid are used, the amounts to add may be determined from the amount and kind of formula and the amount of juice rich in ascorbic acid being consumed by the infant.

Progressive changes should be made in food selection in order to meet the increasing allowances for nutrients. By the age of 12 months the infant should be receiving 3 meals a day. Feedings between meals will probably still be necessary, and may be orange juice or milk.

Diet Plan For the Full Term Infant From 3 to 12 Months of Age

Knowledge of infant nutrition is not complete. However, based on present concepts, a progressive plan for the first year is outlined. Infants vary in their readiness for new foods and different food textures, so the ages indicated should be used only as a rough guide.

Juices, pureed foods, pureed and/or strained milk soups, and soft foods such as mashed potatoes, puddings, and ice cream are included in the infant diet according to the following plan. These foods are given to the infant in addition to the formula. Milk and juices are offered between meals to those infants who are able to drink from a cup.

At 3 months, in addition to the feedings of milk, the infant should have these foods daily:

1. Three ounces orange or grapefruit juice, or at least 4-1/2 ounces tomato juice. The breast-fed infant will not require this

if the mother's intake of ascorbic acid consistently meets recommendations.

2. One or more tablespoons of an iron-containing food as the first solid food. This may be cooked egg yolk, strained meat, or an iron-rich infant cereal.

At about 4 months, in addition to the feedings of milk, the infant should have these foods daily:

1. Three or more ounces orange or grapefruit juice or 5 ounces tomato juice.
2. One or more tablespoons cooked egg yolk, pureed meat, or iron-rich infant cereal.
3. One or more tablespoons pureed fruit.
4. One or more tablespoons pureed vegetables. Dark-green and deep-yellow vegetables are encouraged for frequent use because of their vitamin values.

By about 6 months, in addition to the milk feedings, the infant should have these foods daily:

1. Three or more ounces orange or grapefruit juice or 5 ounces tomato juice.
2. One or more tablespoons infant cereal.
3. One or more tablespoons pureed meat or cooked egg yolk.
4. One or more tablespoons pureed fruit.
5. One or more tablespoons pureed vegetable.
6. Soups, custards, ice cream, puddings, butter or margarine, plain cookies, hard crackers, teething biscuits, or other appropriate additions to the foods listed above.

At about 9 months the baby will probably be eating three meals a day with feedings between meals. He will be ready to eat finely-chopped or junior foods and bread or toast. *NUTS, POPCORN, WHOLE KERNEL CORN, OR OTHER HARD FOODS WHICH MIGHT BE ASPIRATED SHOULD NOT BE GIVEN.* At about this time he should start feeding himself. His diet should progress until it includes the foods listed below as suitable for the year-old child.

At 12 months the baby will still probably require feedings between meals. He will be feeding himself much of his food and probably will be drinking a large portion of his milk from a cup. The diet offered at this age should include each day:

1. Two to 3 cups fortified milk.
2. One egg.
3. One or more tablespoons chopped or junior meat.
4. Two servings (2 to 4 tablespoons is a serving at this age) of soft or junior vegetables. Every other day one of these servings should be a dark-green or deep-yellow vegetable. One serving may be potato.
5. Three or more ounces orange or grapefruit juice or fruit, or other juice that is a good source of ascorbic acid.
6. Two small servings, 1 to 2 tablespoons each, of a soft or junior fruit. Portions can be increased to 3 to 4 tablespoons each.
7. Three slices bread or 2 slices bread and 1 serving cereal.

FOOD FOR TODDLERS:
CHILDREN ONE TO THREE YEARS OLD

This diet is planned for children aged from one to three years for whom no dietary restrictions or special additions of food are indicated. It continues the education of the infant in the colors, odors, flavors, and textures of the variety of foods in this world. Attention in planning this diet is given to these considerations:

1. The mechanism of swallowing is established but the child is learning how much food to take as a bite and how to manage it skillfully in his mouth. Large pieces of any food are not provided, and sticky substances are avoided.

2. The taste buds at this age are particularly sensitive to irritating materials and strong flavors.

3. The teeth and jaws are developing. Some food that requires chewing is included in each meal.

4. The child is learning to feed himself; foods that may be managed easily with fingers, fork, or spoon are provided.

5. He is conservative in taste, and does not appreciate mixtures of different kinds of foods. Vegetables, fruit, eggs, and tender meats are served plain. Combined foods are simple desserts such as custard, milk or fruit puddings, plain cake or cookies, ice cream. Fruit may be served raw in convenient pieces or cooked with a small amount of sugar.

Food Plan

The general diet is the starting point for planning this diet. The menus are not restricted in the number of items served but the portions are small. In this way variety is provided for the child's meals.

Sizes of servings increase gradually and vary according to the appetite. At three years servings will be 1/4 to 1/2 cup in size.

Simple salads and desserts, raw vegetable sticks or fruit sections are included in this diet. Fried foods and foods that are concentrated in sweets or seasonings are omitted, as are vegetables and fruit with high fiber content.

Foods unfamiliar to the child may be offered to him in a hospital. Acceptance of these foods may be sporadic and unpredictable and should be treated with patience.

Daily Plan for Hospital Diet for Toddlers

Milk Group

Two cups fortified whole milk, plus about 1/2 cup more in soups, puddings, or ice cream.

Meat Group

Meat, fish, poultry, eggs. Four to 4-1/2 ounces divided among the three meals. The usual pattern is 2 ounces at noon, 1-1/2 ounces at night; egg (3/week) or strip of crisp bacon at breakfast, or cereal with milk.

Vegetable-Fruit Group

Five servings, including: one serving vitamin C food daily, 1 serving dark-green or deep-yellow vegetable every other day, 3 to 4 servings other vegetables or fruit.

Bread-Cereal Group

Whole grain, enriched, or fortified. One serving of cereal a day. One-half to 1 slice of bread, or 1 graham cracker at a meal.

Fats and Oils

Three pats of butter in the day; each pat about 1/5 ounce.

Sugar

One-half teaspoon sugar was included in the calculations.

Combined Foods

One or 2 simple desserts such as a cooky, pudding, or ice cream. Ingredients may include foods from the foregoing dietary recommendations; if so, they are counted toward the day's total. Other ingredients may be fats, sugar, refined cereal, flour.

Note: Nuts, popcorn, whole kernel corn, or other hard foods which might be aspirated should not be given. Foods offered between meals should have good nutritional value. *Empty calorie* foods such as pop and candy dull the appetite for more nutritious foods. Life-time habits in relation to food are being established during the early years of life.

FOOD FOR CHILDREN AND YOUNG PEOPLE

This diet is planned for children over three years of age, and is suitable for all children and young people for whom no dietary restrictions or special food additions are indicated and for whom no modification in food texture is required.

Diet Plan

The hospital general diet is planned to be *middle-of-the-road* in respect to seasonings, fried foods, concentrated sweets, and foods with a large amount of fiber. Little change is made accordingly for children. Sandwiches, well-liked by most children, are included in the planned menus and as an alternate selection.

There is a wide range in the amount of food ingested by pre-school and school age children and adolescents. The number of items in these menus is kept the same for all ages; the sizes of the servings are increased according to age and appetite but not beyond a sensible amount for the teenagers. The increased requirements of the adolescent are met by generous servings at meals, and additional foods of good nutritive value in between-meal feedings.

Older children are more experienced in their acquaintance with foods, and more venturesome in trying new ones. However, food mixtures such as casserole combinations, frequently rejected by them, are included only occasionally in the hospital menus. Foods such as pizza, french-fried potatoes with ketchup, and well-seasoned sausages may be included at times for them. *Empty calorie* foods such as sweetened beverages are not included unless the fluid intake must be increased and other fluids are rejected by the child.

Daily Plan for Hospital General Diet for Children
Over Three Years of Age

Milk Group
Three cups fortified whole milk, plus about 1/4 cup more in

soups, puddings, ice cream or the equivalent in cheese.

Meat Group

Meat, fish, poultry, eggs, and the alternates, dry beans and peas, nuts, peanut butter. Six ounces divided among the three meals. The usual pattern is 3 ounces (cooked weight) at one meal, 2 ounces at another, and 1 egg or 1 ounce of meat at breakfast occasionally instead of cereal.

Vegetable-Fruit Group

Five to 5-1/2 servings, including: one vitamin C food daily, 1 dark-green or deep-yellow vegetable every other day. Three to 4 servings of other vegetables or fruit every day.

Bread-Cereal Group

Four servings, whole-grain, enriched, or fortified. Usual pattern is 1 serving cereal during the day and 1 slice of bread at each of

TABLE II-3

CALCULATED NUTRIENT ESTIMATES OF GENERAL DIETS FOR INFANTS

| Nutrients | Unit | Recommended Dietary Allowances For Infant 2 to 6 Months | Hospital Diet for Infant 3/12 Months | | |
			(a) Food Other Than Milk	(b) 2 Cups Fortified Milk	Totals (a + b)
Food energy	Calorie	kg x 117 or lb x 53	603	340	945
Protein	gm	kg x 2.2 or lb x 1 gm	29	16	45
Fat	gm	—	18	20	38
Carbohydrate	gm	—	79	24	103
Calcium	gm	0.36	0.3	0.6	0.9
Phosphorus	gm	0.24	0.4	0.5	0.9
Iron	mg	10.0	10.5	—	10.5
Magnesium	mg	60.0	86.5	63.5	150.0
Sodium	mg	—	836.0	244.0	1,066.0
Sodium mEq			36.0	10.0	46.0
Potassium	mg	—	1,078.0	703.0	1,781.0
Potassium mEq			28.0	18.0	46.0
Vitamin A	IU	1,400	4,698	683	5,381
Vitamin D	IU	400	—	200.0	200
Vitamin E		4 IU	1.6 mg	0.3 mg	1.9 mg
Ascorbic acid	mg	35.0	68.0	5.0	73.0
Folacin	mg	0.05	—	—	—
Niacin	mg	5.0	13.3	3.2	16.5
Riboflavin	mg	0.4	0.7	0.8	1.5
Thiamin	mg	0.3	0.7	0.1	0.8
Vitamin B$_6$	mg	0.3	0.6	0.2	0.8
Vitamin B$_{12}$	mcg	0.3	1.2	2.0	3.2

Diet in Health and Disease

the three meals. Occasional use is made of other grain products such as crackers, noodles, rice, macaroni.

Fats and Oils

Three pats of butter a day.

Sugar

One teaspoon sugar (1 packet) was included each day in the calculations.

Combined Foods

One to 2 servings in a day. These include the ice cream and puddings mentioned in the Milk Group as well as cookies, sherbet, cake. Ingredients may include foods from the other basic food groups; if so, they are counted toward the day's total. Additional ingredients may be fats, sugar, refined cereals, flour.

Desserts offered to the younger children are simple puddings,

TABLE II-4

CALCULATED NUTRIENT ESTIMATES OF DIETS FOR CHILDREN

Nutrients	Unit	Recommended Dietary Allowances		Hospital General Diet	
		Children, 1-3 Years	Children, 7-10 Years	Children, 1-3 Years	Children Over 3 Years
Food energy	Calorie	1,300	2,400	1,445	2,185
Protein	gm	23	36	60	105
Fat	gm	—	—	65	85
Carbohydrate	gm	—	—	150	260
Calcium	gm	0.8	0.8	1.0	1.4
Phosphorus	gm	0.8	0.8	1.3	1.7
Iron	mg	15.0	10.0	17.0	15.0
Magnesium	mg	150.0	250.0	172.0	307.0
Sodium	mg	—	—	1,837.0	4,049.0
Sodium mEq				80.0	176.0
Potassium	mg	—	—	2,366.0	3,394.0
Potassium mEq				61.0	87.0
Vitamin A	IU	2,000	3,300	5,866	9,148
Vitamin D*	IU	400	400	200	300
Vitamin E		7 IU	10 IU	3.2 mg	4.8 mg
Ascorbic acid	mg	40.0	40.0	77.0	88.0
Folacin	mg	0.1	0.3	—	—
Niacin	mg	9.0	16.0	24.0	32.0
Riboflavin	mg	0.8	1.2	1.9	2.7
Thiamin	mg	0.7	1.2	1.0	1.6
Vitamin B$_6$	mg	0.6	1.2	1.2	1.8
Vitamin B$_{12}$	mcg	1.0	2.0	4.4	6.7

*Vitamin D provided by fortified milk: 2 cups for the child from 1 to 3 years; 3 cups for the child over three years.

custards, plain cake, and cookies. Those for the adolescent may be more elaborate. One or more of the desserts may be omitted, and a fruit substituted for a reduction in calories.

Between-meal servings may be a milkshake, milk with a sandwich, an apple and crackers, fruit juice and a cookie, ice cream.

REFERENCES

Adults

Balsley, M; Brink, MF; Speckmann, EW: Nutrition in disease and stress. *Geriatrics, 26*:89, Mar, 1971.

Brown, RR: Normal and pathological conditions which may alter the human requirement for vitamin B_6. *Agric Food Chem, 20*:494, 1972.

Finch, CA: Iron metabolism. *Nutr Today, 4*:2, Summer 1969.

Howell, SC; Loeb, MB: Nutrition and aging—a monograph for practitioners. *Gerontologist, 9*:1, Part II, Number 3, 1969.

Irwin, MS; Hegsted, DM: A conspectus of research on amino acid requirements of man. *J Nutr, 101*:539, 1971.

Joint FAO/WHO Expert Committee on Protein Requirements: *Protein Requirements.* FAO Nutr Meet Report Ser No 37; WHO Tech Report Ser No 301, Rome, 1965.

Koch, JP; Donaldson, RK: A survey of food intolerances in hospitalized patients. *N Engl J Med, 271*:657, 1964.

National Academy of Sciences—National Research Council, Food and Nutrition Board: *Recommended Dietary Allowances,* 8th ed, 1974.

Romo, GS; Linkswiler, H: Effect of level and pattern of essential amino acids on nitrogen retention of adult man. *J Nutr, 97*:147, 1969.

Rose, WC: The amino acid requirements of adult man. *Nutr Abst & Rev, 27*:631, 1957.

Van Itallie, TB (Moderator): Conference on the American diet: Healthy or hazardous? *Bull NY Acad Med, 47*:606, 1971.

Pregnancy and Lactation

Arena, JM: Contamination of the ideal food. *Nutr Today, 5*:2, Winter, 1970.

Guthrie, HA: Nutrition in pregnancy and lactation. In Guthrie, HA: *Introductory Nutrition,* 2nd ed. St Louis, Mosby, 1971, Chap 16.

Hillman, RW; Goodhart, RS: Nutrition in pregnancy. In Goodhart, RS; Shils, ME (Eds.): *Modern Nutrition in Health and Disease,* 5th ed. Philadelphia, Lea & Febiger, 1973, Chap 23.

Macy, IG; Kelly, HJ: Food for expectant and nursing mothers. In *Food: The Yearbook of Agriculture.* Washington, DC, USDA, 1959.

Natl Acad Sci—Natl Res Council, Committee on Maternal Nutrition: *Maternal Nutrition and the Course of Pregnancy.* Washington, DC, NAS-NRC, 1970.

Pike, R; Gursky, DD: Further evidence of the deleterious effects produced by sodium restriction during pregnancy. *Am J Clin Nutr, 23*:883, 1970.

Shank, RE: A chink in our armor. *Nutr Today, 5*:2, Summer, 1970. This is a review of the 1970 publication *Maternal Nutrition and the Course of Pregnancy* by NAS-NRC.

Winick, M: Fetal malnutrition and growth processes. *Hosp Practice, 5*:33, May, 1970.

Infants, Toddlers, and Youth

American Academy of Pediatrics, Committee on Nutrition: On the feeding of solid foods to infants. *Pediatrics, 21*:685, 1958.

————: Proposed changes in Food and Drug regulations concerning formula products and vitamin-mineral supplements for infants. *Pediatrics, 40*:916, 1967.

————: Nutritional management of hereditary metabolic disease. *Pediatrics, 40*:289, 1967.

Barnett, HL (in collaboration with Einhorn, AH): *Pediatrics,* 14th ed. New York, Appleton-Century-Crofts, 1968.

Berenberg, W; Mandell, F; Fellers, FX: Hazards of skimmed milk, unboiled and boiled. *Pediatrics, 44*:734, 1969.

Chase, HP; Martin, H: Undernutrition and child development. *N Engl J Med, 282*:933, 1970.

Cheek, DB; Graystone, JE; Read, MS: Cellular growth, nutrition, and development. (Review article) *Pediatrics, 45*:315, 1970.

Davidson, M: Formula feeding of normal term and low birth weight infants. *Pediatr Clin North Am, 17*:913, 1970.

Dayton, DH: Early malnutrition and human development. *Children, 16*:211, 1969.

De Luca, HF: Vitamin D. *N Engl J Med, 281*:1103, 1969.

Di Sant', Agnese P; Talamo, R: Pathogenesis and physiopathology of cystic fibrosis of the pancreas. *N Engl J Med, 277*:1287, 1967.

Finberg, L: The management of the critically ill child with dehydration secondary to diarrhea. *Pediatrics, 45*:1029, 1970.

Fomon, SJ: *Infant Nutrition.* Philadelphia, Saunders, 1967.

————; Thomas, LN; Filer, LJ: Acceptance of unsalted strained foods by normal infants. *J Pediatr, 76*:242, 1970.

Fowler, JR: *Handbook of Infant Formulas.* New York, JB Roerig Division, C Pfizer & Co, Inc, 1967.

Francis, DE; Dixon, DJW: *Diets for Sick Children,* 2nd ed. Oxford and Edinburgh, Blackwell Scientific Publications, 1970.

Herbst, JH; Sunshine, P; Kretchmer, NJ: Intestinal malabsorption in infancy and childhood. In Shulman, L (Ed): *Advances in Pediatrics.* Medical Year Book, Chicago, Medical Publishers, Inc., 1969, Vol 16, page 11.

Hill, LF: Artificial feeding of infants. In Kelley, VC (Ed.): *Brennemann's Practice of Pediatrics.* Hagerstown, Md, Hoeber Medical Div of

Harper & Row, 1969, Vol I, Part I, Chap 26.

Holt, KS; Coffey, VP: *Some Recent Advances in Newborn Errors of Metabolism.* Baltimore, Williams & Wilkins, 1968.

Holt, LE, Jr: Amino acid requirements of infants. *Curr Ther Res, 9*:149, 1967.

Johnston, JA: Adolescence. In Kelley, VC (Ed.): *Brennemann's Practice of Pediatrics.* Hagerstown, Hoeber Medical Div. of Harper & Row, 1969, Vol I, Part I, Chap 26.

Knittle, JL: Obesity in childhood: A problem of adipose tissue cellular development. *J Pediatr, 81*:1048, 1972.

Laupus, WE; Bennett, MJ: Nutritional requirements. In Nelson, WE (Ed.); Vaughn, VC III; McKay, RJ (Assoc. Eds.): *Textbook of Pediatrics.* Philadelphia, Saunders, 1969, page 127.

Lowe, CU et al: Iron balance and requirements in infancy. *Pediatrics, 43*:134, 1969.

Lowe, CU: Research on infant nutrition: The untapped well. *Am J Clin Nutr, 25*:245, 1972.

Michener, WM (Ed.): Symposium on gastrointestinal disorders. *Pediatr Clin North Am, 14*:1, 1967.

Owen, GM: Modification of cow's milk for infant formulas: Current practice. *Am J Clin Nutr, 22*:1150, 1969.

Panos, TC; Younathan, MT: Nutritional requirements of infants and children. In Kelley, VC (Ed.): *Brennemann's Practice of Pediatrics.* Hagerstown, Hoeber Medical Div. of Harper & Row, 1969, Vol I, Part I, Chap 23.

Shaw, JH: New knowledge of nutrition and dental caries. *Med Clin North Am, 54*:1555, 1970.

Staff of Dept of Nutrition: *Recent Advances in Therapeutic Diets.* University of Iowa Medical Center, Iowa Univ Press, Iowa City, 1970.

Stanbury, JB; Wyngaarden, JB; Fredrickson, DS (Eds.): *The Metabolic Basis of Inherited Disease,* 3rd ed. New York, McGraw Hill, 1972.

Townley, RR: Management of chronic or recurrent diarrhea in childhood. *Postgrad Med J, 45*:135, Feb, 1969.

Medical Year Book, Chicago, Medical Publishers, Inc, 1969, Vol 16,

US Children's Bureau: Feeding the child with a handicap. USPHS Publ 2091. US Government Printing Office, Washington, DC, 1970.

US Dept of Health, Education, and Welfare: Height and Weight of Children, United States. National Center for Health Statistics, Series 11, No 104. US Govt Printing Office, Washington, DC, 1970.

Winick, M: Cellular growth during early malnutrition. *Pediatrics, 47*:967, 1971.

——— (Ed.): *Nutrition and Development.* New York, Wiley-Interscience, 1972.

Wolman, IF: Some prominent developments in childhood nutrition: 1972. *Clin Pediatr, 12*:72, Feb. 1973.

LIQUID DIETS

I NDIVIDUALS VARY GREATLY in their recovery following tissue injury. The extent of the biological components of the trauma, history of previous illness, and the nutritional state prior to surgery or other tissue injury will influence the rate of recovery. Moore (1967) classifies the scale of traumatic injury in terms of the biological components as follows. These effects are additive.

Minor stimuli such as short term immobilization, lack of food, anesthesia, fear, cold, pain, fatigue, and minor tissue injury. Most body responses to these short term stimuli are small and quickly reversed. Long term stimuli such as would result from immobilization in chronic illnesses, starvation, and infection are resistant to reversal.

Threatening challenges such as plasma volume loss, blood volume loss, desalting, dehydration, traumatic edema, hypotension, anoxia, hypercarbia, and major tissue injury.

Tissue-necrosing trauma such as sepsis, gangrene, shock, and extensive tissue injury. These result in necrotic or anoxic tissue in the body for a long time. Infections are a strong stimulus to compositional and endocrine changes. Prolonged shock involves a deficiency of flow of body fluids resulting in biochemical alterations. Necrotic tissue is a threat to the kidneys. In addition to these non-endocrine bodily changes after trauma, there are endocrine responses which greatly affect metabolism.

Moore divides surgical convalescence into four phases:

1. A phase of injury characterized by a loss of lean tissue and fat from the body, and a relative gain in body water and the extracellular components. The patient rarely has an appetite for food at this time.

2. A turning point during which there is a reduction in the absolute urinary nitrogen rate, a return of peristalsis, and a desire for food. During this phase diuresis is usually present. The first and second phases in uncomplicated surgery generally do not last more than a day or two each following surgery. In case of infections the period may be extended. Food, even if tolerated, will not reverse the tissue catabolism. Fluids are essential.
3. A period of spontaneous nitrogen anabolism with a return to pre-injury body mass and with recovery of strength. Adequate nutrient intake is essential during this period.
4. A period of redeposition of fat to former levels.

The physician orders the progression from clear to full liquids and then to a more general diet. The importance of the nutrients provided for the convalescent cannot be over-rated. Vitamin C, protein, zinc, and magnesium influence the rate of wound healing. Trace elements are a part of a number of enzyme systems concerned with tissue metabolism. Supplementation is recommended.

A clear liquid diet of non-residue foods provides fluids, certain electrolytes including potassium, and some calories chiefly from carbohydrates. Chemically defined diets of synthetic non-residue nutrients have been developed commercially. These include known nutrients and micronutrients in elemental form.

Gastrointestinal distress, frequently caused by gas, is a common complaint following trauma. See section on "Flatulence," Appendix I. Note especially the references concerning the influence of fruit juice selection, and drugs, on gas production.

Full liquid diets traditionally have been composed of conventional foods. Commercial processors have recently developed products that are combinations of foods and elemental nutrients. See sections following.

CLEAR LIQUID DIET

Clear liquids are offered as soon as tolerated, and include those clear foods that are liquid or that will liquify at body temperatures. Foods included:
Broth, consomme
Clear tea, coffee, decaffeinated beverage
Carbonated beverages: 7-Up, gingerale
Apple and grape juice with added vitamin C, pineapple juice,

juices of canned or cooked fruits. Drinks made with fruit-flavored granules with vitamin C added. Avoid prune juice. Clear gelatin desserts made with water or canned fruit juice, jello
Salt, sugar. Extremes of sugar and salt are to be avoided
Meal Pattern, clear liquid diet:
Liquids are offered at the regular meal times and as between-meal feedings. For example:

		Quantity	
		cc	Measure
Morning	Apple juice with added vitamin C	120	1/2 cup
	Gelled fruit or vegetable juice	120	1/2 cup
	Coffee or tea, sugar	240	1 cup
Noon	Broth, chicken or beef	120	1/2 cup
	Fruit juice	120	1/2 cup
	Gelled fruit or vegetable juice	120	1/2 cup
Night	Broth	240	1 cup
	Fruit juice	120	1/2 cup
	Popsicle	120	1/2 cup
	Total	1440cc	6 cups

Between meal feedings mid-morning and mid-afternoon of about one cup each will bring the quantity of fluid to about 2000 cc. These feedings may be carbonated beverages, fruit drinks or juices, broth, tea or coffee with sugar. Orange juice is thought by some physicians to cause distress after certain surgical procedures and should not be included except with physician approval during the period that a patient is on clear liquids.

The minimal water requirement of average individuals was given by the National Research Council in 1968 and is quoted in Section I. For the average well adult this amounts to 2000-3000 ml, of which about one-half is lost through vaporization and one-half is excreted as urine.

The fluid requirement of the post-operative patient is influenced by many factors. It is to be expected that he will not ingest all that he is offered. The physician will order if fluids are to be increased beyond the quantities listed in the clear liquid meal pattern. In cases of renal or cardiac insufficiency, fluids may need to be decreased.

FULL LIQUID DIET

The full liquid diet, which is essentially the same as the Smooth Diet, Section III, consists of foods that are of 'pour' consistency or that are liquid at body temperature. This diet should be planned to include the foods in the basic food groups. For the person with chronic disease who must live on this diet for a long time particular attention should be directed to increasing the quantities of the basic foods. Weight and blood chemistry should be observed closely.

Following is a detailed description of the full liquid or smooth diet; in Section III is a list of some of the conditions in which a smooth diet is suitable. The full liquid diet includes all of the foods in the clear liquid diet plus the following:

Milk Group

Whole, skim, low fat milk, buttermilk, yogurt, cream, evaporated milk. Cocoa, chocolate milk, eggnog made with pasteurized mix. Cream (milk) soups. Ice cream, sherbet, custards, soft puddings.

Meat Group

Lean meats cooked and blenderized (pureed) with broth to liquify. Stock soups with strained vegetables. Homogenized baby meats with cereal gruels.

Vegetables and Fruits

Vegetable and fruit juices. May be gelled. Pureed vegetables are accepted best in soups. Soft-cooked fruits strained with added juice to liquify.

Cereals

Milk toast (crust removed), cereal gruels with milk, cream, or fruit juice.

Fats, Sugars

As desired and as tolerated. May be added when increased calories are needed. Brown sugar has higher potassium than white.

Meal Pattern, full liquid or smooth diet:

Foods are offered six times a day; usually three items at meal periods, and one or two items between meals and at night.

	Example	Alternate Selection
Morning	Fruit juice, any kind	Orange juice is included
	Cereal gruel with	Instant farina, quick

	Example	Alternate Selection
	milk or cream	rolled oats
	Coffee or tea	
	with sugar and cream	
Mid-morning	Milk or malted	May be flavored with
	milk shake	Kool-Aid
Noon	Tomato juice	Or V-8 juice
	Cream of pea soup	Or other strained
		vegetable soup
	Vanilla ice cream	Or smooth sherbet
Afternoon	Fruit juice	Apple or grape juice with
		vitamin C added
	Yogurt or eggnog	
Evening	Fruit drink	
	Cereal gruel with milk	Butter may be added
	Cocoa or other beverage	
Night	Carbonated beverage	Added ice cream will
		increase calories
		and protein

To promote appetite, liquids of low osmolal concentration are a good choice. Extremes of sugar and salt are to be avoided but fats may be moderately increased.

A milk-free liquid diet may be ordered for the person who has an intolerance for milk. The medical basis for the restriction of milk and milk products will determine the selection of other sources of protein. If *no* milk products are tolerated, soy milk may be useful. Additional blenderized or homogenized meats would be included, and the chemically defined liquid supplements may be used as outlined following. If *lactose* must be limited, small amounts of fermented milks (buttermilk, yogurt) may be allowed if consumed with other foods. Aged cured cheese can be added to soups. A lactose-free liquid diet is outlined in Section VI, and the lactose content of some common foods is listed.

With losses in food processing and the increased nutrient demand in chronic disease where the selection and quantity ingested may be limited, vitamin and mineral supplementation may be wise if the liquid diet is the sole source of nutrition for some time. Formula feedings and synthetic oral feedings are being widely used.

TUBE FEEDINGS

The following qualities are desirable in tube feedings. They should:

1. Contain all essential nutrients and micronutrients in quantities and ratios needed to maintain or achieve normal blood levels.
2. Approximate the average diet in ratios of calories:

      12 to 20% in protein

      25 to 50% in fat

      40 to 50% in carbohydrate

The above ratios should result in a suitable protein-calorie ratio. Carbohydrates frequently included are maltose, lactose, dextrose, dextrin, and modified starches. Sucrose improves palatability if the same product is to be used as an oral feeding. Polyunsaturated fats have been used in some formulas.
3. Have a known, easily calculated nutrient value. One calorie per milliliter of product has been widely used.
4. *Not* be highly concentrated. High electrolyte and high protein concentrations, if not accompanied by adequate water administration, may result in high serum and urinary osmolality leading to high blood urea nitrogen (BUN) and dehydration. An average American diet ranges between 500 and 600 milliosmols per liter (private communication).
5. Be sterile, if canned, pasteurized if home prepared.
6. Be homogenized for easy flow through a small caliber tube.
7. Be packaged in quantities suitable for administration over a limited period of time to control bacterial hazards.
8. Be refrigerated after opening if not administered immediately.

Early tube feedings were modifications of eggnog prepared in the institution as needed. These were made with higher concentrations of milk solids than regular milk or cream. They were high in osmolal concentration. Prior to use of pasteurized egg products, salmonella contamination was a constant hazard.

This type of formula with added essential fatty acids, minerals, and vitamins, but without egg was developed and is currently on the market as a dry powder (such as Sustagen, Meritene) and as a canned liquid such as Meritene Liquid®, Metrecal®, Sego®, Instant Breakfast®, Slender®, etc. The liquid canned formulas were promoted originally for low calorie diets and for quick complete meals, recently as dietary supplements and for short term total nourishment. Newer products of similar composition are being promoted for tube feedings. They are high in protein, carbohydrate and osmolal concentration.

Sustacal® (Mead Johnson) was put on the market in 1971. It contains concentrated skim milk, sugar, soy oil, sodium casseninate, corn syrup solids, and minerals and vitamins. It is 55% carbohydrate, 24% protein, and 21% fat.

Nutri-1000® (Syntax Laboratories, Inc), announced in 1972, contains skim milk, sucrose, soy oil, coconut oil, dextrin-maltose-dextrose, minerals and vitamins. It contains 40% carbohydrate, 13% protein, and 47% fat.

Most of these fortified milk products are high in electrolytes and osmolal concentration.

During the 1950's blenderized "whole meal" feedings came into use. They include milk, meats, cereal, vegetables, and fruit juice selected for nutritional value and can be formulated to meet the recommended nutritional allowances for specific individuals. They approximate the proportion of carbohydrate, protein, and fat in the average American diet. They have finely divided fiber of value for peristalsis and are relatively low in osmolal concentration. Frequently they are supplemented with minerals which change the osmolal concentration.

In the institutional preparation of this kind of feeding, homogenized meats, vegetables, and fruits sold as baby foods ease the preparation. Homogenized meat-base baby formulas and homogenized meat-cereal-vegetable mixtures may be used to achieve a stable mixture which will not clog the feeding tube. However, use of these finely divided, highly processed products opens a question as to nutrient losses.

If liver and/or pasteurized egg powder are used in the feedings the inclusion of unsaturated vegetable oils will help avoid increased cholesterol levels in the blood.

Evaporated milk may be used as an ingredient. It is homogenized and sterilized and contains vitamin D.

Aseptic technique should be observed in the preparation, handling, and administration of all feedings. Terminal sterilization is desirable.

A rotation of foodstuffs to provide variety within each food group is good practice in long continued use. Formulas composed of basic foodstuffs have been published. These can be adapted to specific nutrient needs. See textbooks by Goodhart and Shils (1973), Robinson, (1972), and the diet manuals listed in the general references, Appendix IV, for formulas.

Problems may be encountered in institutional preparation of tube feedings:

Preparation time is expensive and much supervision is required.

Although most institutions have blenders, practically none have homogenizers. The non-homogenized product separates and clogs the small tube used for administration.

Means to sterilize the containers and to pasteurize or sterilize the product may not be readily available.

Control of time and temperature in the distribution and administration of a non-sterile product may not be ideal.

In the early 1970's formulas containing common foodstuffs fortified with minerals and vitamins were developed as canned feedings as outlined above.

The carbohydrate content of these products is lower than that of the earlier formulas which were chiefly milk and milk solids. Osmolal concentration varies from product to product ranging from about 600 to 2000 milliosmols per liter or more.

Pharmacies will provide information on products marketed at this time. Most are advertised in the Journal of the American Dietetic Association.

Formulas of compounded foods are changed as clinical experience and nutritional knowledge warrants. Current analysis should be obtained before use.

When a formula feeding provides the total nutrition it is of the utmost importance that a record of total daily intake of formula and additional water be maintained.

CHEMICALLY DEFINED (ELEMENTAL) DIETS

Stimulated by the need for food for men in space, Winitz et al (1965) developed a diet of chemically discrete components. This was composed of glucose, *L*-amino acids, ethyl linoleate, minerals, and vitamins. This formula has been adapted to medical use.

This chemically defined diet, now termed "elemental diet," contains known elements for nutritional support at a level of one calorie per milliliter. Its use results in a reduction of microflora populations in the gut, and less frequent and smaller than average bowel movements (Winitz et al, 1970).

Research is continuing on its use in various catabolic states. Stephens and Randall (1969) report success with the elemental diet in patients unable to tolerate conventional foodstuffs, or whose intake is inadequate. See references following for recommendations and evaluations of practices in parenteral nutrition.

Several groups have questioned the adequacy of Rose's standard for essential amino acids. Weller, Calloway and Mergen found it to be inadequate for their subjects. They found amino acids in concentration and ratios appearing in a hydrolysate of native egg white to be superior to Rose's mixture.

The osmolality of chemically formulated diets is high. Feedings should always be given slowly. Further dilution may be required. When used either as an oral or a tube feeding additional water should always be given and the patient monitored for signs of dehydration and electrolyte imbalance (Gault, 1968).

At this time (1973) chemically formulated liquid diets are available from Eaton Laboratories through pharmacies: Vivonex-100® is a chemically defined water soluble elemental diet in six flavors. This is described by the manufacturer as a standard diet and contains 1.22% available nitrogen in the form of pure amino acids. Vivonex-100 HN® is an elemental *high* nitrogen diet providing 2.5% available nitrogen.

Both of these Vivonex formulas are bulk-free. They are provided in single-feeding packets of soluble powder which, when diluted as recommended, may be used for drinking or as a tube feeding. However they lack palatability for long-continued oral use. The manufacturer recommends that they be used only under a physician's supervision and suggests their use as a tube feeding, as a clear liquid diet, and when minimal intestinal contents is an objective in the care of the patient.

These products are high in osmolal concentration; specific directions (provided with the material) should be observed to avoid complications such as diarrhea or gastrointestinal distress. Additional fluids should be provided.

At the present time (1973) Vivonex-100® costs considerably more than calorie equivalent portions of the milk-base formulas. The high nitrogen product (Vivonex-100 HN®) is even more expensive.

Other pharmaceutical houses are developing low residue oral feedings. Local pharmacies will be able to provide information on them. Greenfield and Briggs (1971) point out the frequency with which purified diets have been found deficient in certain nutrients although described by the supplier as being complete. A lack of mention of level of use was also evident. Although the study concerned mixtures for rats, precautions mentioned by the authors are worthy of note in the use of purified mixtures for human nutrition under conditions of stress.

Precautions in the use of tube feedings:
The patient's head should be elevated if a semi-upright position is not possible.

Water should be supplied in addition to the tube feedings. Fluid intake and output should be monitored.

In initiating a regimen of tube feedings, the starting amounts should be small in quantity and may be diluted with sterile water to produce a less concentrated mixture. Several days may be required for a patient to adjust to the feeding. Increase to adequate caloric intake should be gradual.

Feedings by tube should be given slowly, preferably by drip or pump, throughout most of the day.

Diarrhea has been a problem in the use of some liquid feedings taken either orally or by tube. Causes may be bacterial contamination, too rapid administration, improper placement of the tube, feedings too cold, or osmolal concentration too high.

There is danger in assuming that use of a pre-packaged formula feeding ensures meeting the patient's nutrient needs. Most patients on tube feedings in hospitals and nursing homes have suffered nutritional depletion and have impaired absorption and retention. Nutritional status is time related. Careful surveillance of quantities of formula consumed and total daily nutrient intake, with periodic clinical evaluation, is essential. Clinical monitoring is especially needed when administering formulas fortified with amino acids and electrolytes. Dehydration, amino acid imbalances, and toxic reactions can develop rapidly when the patient's normal appetite control is by-passed.

There is a temptation to simply manipulate the quantity of formula to control calories, without assessing the impact of change in volume on amino acid, mineral, and vitamin intake. When the volume consumed is reduced, special supplementation may be needed. Clinical and laboratory findings should indicate such need. Some groups are questioning the wisdom of the very high protein (20% of calories or more) low fat formulas (private communication). Fat supplies needed calories without influencing the osmolal concentration of the formula. Advantages to a low fat (20 to 30% of calories) have not been proven. A formula of 40 to 45% of the calories from fat and 12 to 15 % from protein would more closely approximate the average American diet.

Rather than seeking the "one best" formula, a rotating daily use of several formulas composed of foods from different animal and vegetable products should be considered. By this means a deficiency in any one formula might be corrected by the other formula. Imbalances would be less likely to be long continued.

PARENTERAL ALIMENTATION

Dudrick, Wilmore, and associates (1968) developed *as a surgical procedure* a system for "parenteral hyperalimentation" with a laboratory formulated synthetic diet. They infuse a hypertonic nutrient solution into the superior vena cava, thus allowing rapid dilution and distribution of nutrients. By this method they have given 2000 to 3500 calories in a 24 hour period. Metabolic response to this mode of alimentation has been good, both as a source of total nutrition, and as an adjunct to limited oral intake.

Stegink and Besten (1972) note a need to re-define "essential" and "non-essential" amino acids when the gut is by-passed in alimentation. The gut controls the rate of entry of individual amino acids thereby maintaining normal ratios in the blood and influencing the length of time they are available. These authors note that peptides appear to be absorbed from the gut more rapidly than their component amino acids. Toxicity and amino acid imbalances following direct infusion of amino acids into the bloodstream can cause problems.

Nasset (1972) noted that amino acids can no longer be considered the "innocuous compounds" we have considered them to be, "except in combinations as encountered in normal digestion and metabolism." He points out that pellagra can be produced by adding leucine to a low protein diet; force feeding a low protein diet with the addition of an imbalanced amino acid mixture can lead to pathological conditions.

REFERENCES

American Medical Assoc: *Symposium on Total Parenteral Nutrition.* Chicago, American Medical Assoc, 1972.

Artz, CP; Moncrief, J: *Treatment of Burns.* Philadelphia, Saunders, 1969.

Barnes, BJ: Magnesium conservation: A study of surgical patients. *Ann NY Acad Sci, 162* (art 2):786, 1969.

Calloway, DH; Murphy, EL: Postoperative distension and fruit juice. *JAMA, 194*:476, 1965.

Crews, ER: *Practical Manual for Treatment of Burns,* 2nd ed. Springfield, Thomas, 1967.

Cuthbertson, D: Intensive care—metabolic response to injury. *Brit J Surg, 57*:718, 1970.

————; Tilstone, WJ: Nutrition of the injured. *Am J Clin Nutr, 21*:911, 1968.

Dudrick, SJ; Wilmore, DW; Vars, HM; Rhoads, JE: Long term parenteral nutrition with growth, development, and positive nitrogen balance. *Surgery, 64*:134, July, 1968.

————; Wilmore, DW: Long term parenteral feeding. *Hosp Practice, 3*:65, Oct, 1968.

————; Ruberg, RL: Principles and practice of parenteral nutrition. *Gastroenterol, 61*:901, 1971.

Fatal hyperalimentation syndrome. *Nutr Rev, 35*:121, 1972.

Gault, MH, et al: Hypernatremia, azotemia, and dehydration due to high protein tube feeding. *Ann Intern Med, 68*:778, 1968.

Glotzer, DJ: Space diets. *Gastroenterol, 61*:405, 1971. (Comments on reports of use of chemically defined diets, their advantages and limitations.)

Gormican, A: Inorganic elements in foods used in hospital menus. *J Am Diet Assoc, 56*:397, 1970.

————; Catli, E: Mineral balance in young men fed a fortified milk-base formula. *Nutr Metab, 13*:364, 1971.

————: Nutritional and chemical responses of immobilized patients to a sterile milk-base feeding. *J Chron Dis, 25*:291, 1972.

————; Liddy, E: Tube feedings: Practical considerations in prescription and evaluation. *Postgrad Med, 53*:71, June, 1973.

Greenfield, H; Briggs, GA: Nutritional methodology in metabolic research with rats. *Ann Rev Biochem, 40*:549, 1971.

Hutchin, P: Metabolic response to surgery in relation to calorie, fluid and electrolyte intake. *Curr Probl Surg, 1-51,* Apr, 1971.

Johnson, CL; McIlrath, DC: Management of patients with enterocutaneous fistulas. *Surg Clin North Am, 29*:967, 1969.

Kukral, JC; Shoemaker, WC: Metabolic sequelae of burn trauma. *Surg Clin North Am, 51*:1211, 1970.

Moore, FD: Metabolic response to injury. In Randall, HT; Hardy, JD; Moore, FD (Eds.): *Manual of Preoperative and Postoperative Care.* Philadelphia, Saunders, 1967, Chap 4.

————: Getting well: The biology of surgical convalescence. *Ann NY Acad Sci, 73* (art 2):389, 1958.

Nasset, ES: Amino acid homeostasis in the gut lumen and its nutritional significance. *World Rev Nutr Diet, 14*:134, 1972.

Ohlson, MA: *Experimental and Therapeutic Dietetics,* 2nd ed. Minneapolis, Burgess, 1972.

Pories, WJ, et al: Acceleration of wound healing in man with zinc sulfate given by mouth. *Lancet, 1*:121, 1967.

Porter, R; Knight, J (Eds.): *Energy Metabolism and Trauma. A Ciba Foundation Symposium.* London, J & H Churchhill, 1970.

Rhoads, JE, et al: *Surgery: Principles and Practice,* 4th ed. Philadelphia, Lippincott, 1970, Chap 5 & 6

Shils, ME: Guidelines for total parenteral nutrition. *JAMA, 220*:1721, 1972 and (correction) *221*:1506, 1972.

Stegink, L; Besten, LD: Synthesis of cysteine from methionine in normal adult subjects: Effect of route of alimentation. *Science, 178*:514, 1972.

Stephens, RV; Randall, HT: Use of concentrated balanced liquid elemental diet for nutritional management of catabolic states. *Ann Surg, 170*:642, 1969.

Taylor, WH: Clinical aspects of the metabolic response to trauma. *Am J Clin Nutr, 3*:181, 1955.

Walker, WF; Johnston, IDA: *The Metabolic Basis of Surgical Care.* Philadelphia, Davis, 1971.

Weller, LA; Calloway, DH; Margen, S: Nitrogen balance of men fed amino acid mixtures based on Rose's requirements, egg white protein and serum free amino acid patterns. *J Nutr, 101*:1499, 1971

Winitz, M; Seedman, DA; Graff, J: Studies in metabolic nutrition using chemically defined diets. I, Extended feeding of normal adult males. *Am J Clin Nutr, 23*:525, 1970.

Winitz, M; Adams, RF; Seedman, DA; Davis, PN; Jayco, LG; Hamilton, JA: Studies in metabolic nutrition using chemically defined diets. II, Effect on gut microflora population. *Am J Clin Nutr, 23*:546, 1970.

See also the references in Section II, Diets for Adults.

SECTION IV

MODIFICATIONS IN CONSISTENCY OF FOODS*

THE SOFT DIET WITH VARIATIONS
FOR SPECIFIC CONDITIONS

THIS SOFT DIET AIMS to provide foods that require little effort in eating and that are not a challenge to the gastrointestinal tract. Foods are presented in forms that are recognizable and familiar, leaving the ground meats and strained vegetables to the variations of the soft diet that are necessary to meet different abnormal conditions of the alimentary tract.

The soft diet provides a transition from the full liquid diet to the general diet. It serves also as a beginning point for modifications demanded by the disease condition and the pathophysiology at the site. There will be overlapping in the use of the modifications depending upon the relative severity of the disease condition present. These modifications are not presented as a set pattern for dietary prescriptions. Rather, they are offered as a means to classify foods for these variations and to systematize food preparation in group feeding. They are based on observations by physicians in clinical practice and on reports in the literature.

It is recognized that a given patient will have his own individual combination of symptoms, tolerances, and reactions. With an awareness of the reason for prescribing the diet, and of the nutritional requirements of the patient the soft diet may be varied by means of menu selection to provide the modifications listed below and given in detail in this section. Most patients for whom these diets are ordered will have nutrient needs greater than indicated in the RDA for healthy people.

*Consultants: Kenneth Lemmer, MD, Prof of Surgery, John Morrissey, MD, Prof of Medicine, Univ of Wis Medical School

65

TABLE IV-1
SUGGESTED AND SELECTED INSTANCES FOR THE USE OF THE SOFT DIET AND VARIATIONS

Soft Diet	Mechanical Soft Diet	Smooth Diet (Blenderized; Pureed)	Variations of the Soft Diet	
			Bland Diet	*Modified Residue Diets*
Transition between full liquid and general diets	Following eye surgery	After palate or throat surgery or tonsillectomy	In the care of gastric or duodenal ulcer or other peptic disorders when acute or refractory	1. *Low residue* Preparative for X-ray or operative procedure
After physical or severe mental trauma	For persons who have marked difficulty in chewing and swallowing	When cancerous lesions of the mouth, throat, or gastrointestinal tract are present		For a short time following gastrointestinal surgery
In acute infections				
In certain instances of anorexia				
		In esophagitis	When there are cuts or open lesions in the mouth or throat	In treatment of intestinal fistulas during acute stage (diverticulitis)
Following periodontal surgery		When esophageal stricture, tumor, or varices are present		2. *Restricted Shortened Fiber* In stenosis or neurogenic stasis of the lumen
For persons who are: —elderly —debilitated —easily nauseated		In drug toxicity following chemotherapy	In cases of gastric distress caused by extreme flatulence.	In blind loop syndrome
Following a stroke with unilateral facial paralysis		For persons who have difficulty in opening the mouth or in swallowing		In diverticulosis (soft fiber is increased)

Multiple vitamin supplementation is recommended with each diet. The condition of the patient may indicate mineral supplementation also.

electrolytes) are to be avoided. For this reason refined sugars and salty foods are restricted. Diets of high osmolality may cause sudden fluid shifts. Increased peristalsis may follow. Nausea may occur. There may be diarrhea. Small quantities or dilute forms of the same foods may be tolerated.

If nausea occurs during a meal, the feeding should be stopped and fluids offered as promptly as possible. Smaller servings of less concentrated foods should be offered at the next meal.

Hard coatings on deep-fried foods will slow down the penetration of digestive juices and hence retard the digestive process. Home-type skillet cookery with a limited quantity of fat is less apt to create tough coatings. Such foods are generally tolerated and palatable.

The *soft diet* is useful in many situations although it may not always be ordered in the dietary sequence following surgery. The age, physical, and medical condition of the patient will determine the diet required. Generally, this routine will meet the needs of the debilitated person who lacks energy to eat foods that require much chewing. In cases of severe debilitation, use of the *mechanical soft diet* in which meats are ground and softened by the addition of liquid may promote food consumption by decreasing the effort required to chew the food. It is important to allow plenty of time for meals.

1. In condition involving facial paralysis the soft diet is the plan of choice. Following a stroke with unilateral facial and pharyngeal involvement, there may be decreased oral and facial sensations resulting in difficulty in keeping the lips closed. This may lead to excessive drooling. Soft intact foods of the soft diet are more easily ingested than liquids. If there is the added problem of nasal regurgitation, the use of a drinking tube may lessen the difficulty.

2. In advanced multiple sclerosis or parkinson's disease with attendant neuropathy it is important to maintain mobility of the oral structures (the tongue, jaws, lips, and soft palate) even though there is progressive deterioration in the voluntary activity. The patient can call upon the physiological reserves of his motor mechanisms and should be stimulated to do so by providing intact foods of soft texture. As a therapeutic measure foods such as peanut butter, mashed potatoes, and ice

cream cones which will enhance tongue and lip activity should be offered.

3. For the person with cerebral palsy or facial paralysis the degree of disability will determine the extent of modification required to facilitate swallowing. Small quantities of food should be put in the mouth at a time. Even small amounts of liquid cause difficulty with some people and may be managed more easily if gelled. A spoon with a long handle and a small bowl like an iced tea spoon may be helpful when the individual has to be fed.

MECHANICAL SOFT DIET

This soft diet is of particular use in two situations:

1. *For people who lack teeth.* Individuals vary widely in their ability to chew when without teeth, and have divergent attitudes toward the kind of food they want. This diet may also be used for the person who lacks energy to chew. No foods need be denied, unless otherwise indicated, if the patient believes that he can manage it. There have been frequent reports of lack of proper dental care in long term facilities. Good teeth or well-fitting dentures are essential to thorough mastication. A note in the patient's chart will draw attention to the need.

2. *Following eye surgery* it is essential to decrease the amount of chewing. The diet progresses, after cataract surgery, from full liquid on the day of operation to the general diet on the eighth day postoperative. From the second to the seventh day foods are used that require a minimum of facial motion.

Diet Plan

Either the soft diet or the general diet may be used as a basis for the mechanical soft diet, but all foods must be easy to chew and swallow.

Meat is ground after cooking, unless tender.

Foods may be softened by the addition of broth, milk, or fruit juice.

Hard particles such as nuts and firm pieces of raw vegetable are not included.

Toast and crackers are softened, and bread crusts removed for the person who has had eye surgery.

SMOOTH DIET

The smooth diet offers liquid and semi-solid foods that are easily swallowed and require no chewing.

Diet Plan

All solid foods are reduced to a smooth soft consistency. Liquids, and soft foods such as cooked finely-milled cereals, blenderized thick soups, pureed meats and vegetables, gelled juices, soft puddings, custards, and ice cream are included. If the person has open lesions in the mouth or throat, fruit and fruit juices should be bland rather than acid, and temperature of foods should not be too hot or too cold.

If dry foods such as crackers and toast or solid foods such as firm mashed potatoes are included in the menu they should be combined with some liquid before presentation. Dry foods require tongue movement to turn and moisten them in the mouth.

Since a liquid must be added when blenderizing meat to make it the proper consistency, a 50-gram portion of pureed meat is about equal in protein value to 30 grams of cooked meat that is not pureed. The household measure nearest to 50 grams is one-fourth cup; and the five ounces of meat recommended in the daily food guide is converted to one and one-fourth cups of pureed meats. The strained meats marketed as baby foods are suitable for this use. In current practice the terms "strained", "blenderized", and "pureed" are used interchangeably even though they do not represent precisely the same process or finished product.

For long term use care should be taken to include all of the recommendations of the daily food guide for the Milk, Meat, Vegetable-Fruit, and Bread-Cereal groups. Calories can and must be made adequate. Supplementation with ascorbic acid may be necessary.

Special Considerations in the Use of the Smooth Diet

1. *Following tonsillectomy* there are cuts in throat tissue. Mechanical and chemical irritation must be avoided; acid foods are not included. For the short term of care, foods such as milk, gruels,

bland strained soups, custards, soft puddings, and smooth ice cream offer sufficient variety.

2. *For esophagitis* acid or salty foods and those with sharp edges are omitted.

3. *If there is a tumor of the esophagus or esophageal varices* a smooth diet will facilitate swallowing.

4. *After palate or throat surgery* the restrictions of the bland diet in respect to acid and irritating foods should be observed until cuts are healed. The smooth diet is used but sticky or pasty foods should be avoided. The use of the tongue in clearing food from the mouth may be limited and painful.

5. *In conditions due to cancer of the mouth or throat* foods as outlined for palate or throat surgery are appropriate.

6. *When the jaw is broken* the smooth diet or the mechanical soft diet may be served if the person can open his mouth wide enough to use a spoon. Otherwise he may manage better with a full liquid diet or with an appropriate formula feeding.

7. *When symptoms of drug toxicity follow cancer therapy.* Chewing, swallowing, and salivation capabilities are frequently limited. A full liquid or a smooth diet will usually be selected depending upon the patient's condition and his preference for texture. In hospital practice the smooth diet usually includes a wider selection of foods and more varied textures than the full liquid diet.

It is important that the foods not be so concentrated as to induce nausea. Commercially prepared regular soups and soup bases of high electrolyte content are not a wise choice.

BLAND DIET

The bland diet may be described as mild in flavors, texture, and temperature. Although "bland" means mild or non-irritating only, the mouth and throat conditions for which a bland diet is ordered generally require a soft texture also. The soft diet is used as a foundation and it is modified in general as outlined in the following diet plan. Variations in concentration and in selection of foodstuffs should be made according to individual tolerance. Small quantities of foods usually restricted may be well-tolerated if taken with meals.

Little data are available concerning the effect of individual foods or of a mixed diet on gastrointestinal function, contents, or flora. In the past most diets used in gastrointestinal disorders seemed to be based largely on folklore and habit. Customs related to food, and the local food supply, have also influenced the choice of foods for inclusion in any diet.

Food tolerances are highly individual, and certain foodstuffs are incriminated by some people. This quotation is from an abstract in *Gastroenterology, 55*:139, 1968: "Most forms of food intolerance are a characteristic of the individual and are equally common in health and disease." Since positive data supporting exclusion of many incriminated foods are not available, a liberal diet stressing good nutrition is recommended. It seems safe to assume that a person will eliminate a food from his diet if it causes him discomfort; but because a food distresses one or a few persons that does not warrant eliminating it from the diets of those who can tolerate it. See discussion of "flatulence", pages 232 and 244.

Assurance and supportive direction on the part of the physician and other professional personnel are important adjuncts in therapy.

A relaxed and quiet atmosphere at mealtimes is desirable.

Diet Plan

The bland diet described here is appropriate for hospital or home use and, unless limited by individual desires, will meet the requirements of the recommended dietary allowances.

The dietary modifications required depend on the area affected, the severity of the symptoms, and the patient's general condition. The diet is progressed, when required, from liquid to semi-solid to solid foods. Feedings may begin at 2-hour intervals and advance to the person's usual pattern of meals. The present concept of treatment is toward liberalization of the diet as soon as symptoms abate.

Regularity of mealtimes is important.

Food should be well-chewed, not bolted, but eaten in a relaxed, leisurely manner.

Foods included in the bland diet are:

Milk: whole, skim, or partially skimmed; cream, ice cream; cottage, cream, and plain natural or processed cheeses. Overemphasis of milk to the exclusion of other foods is to be avoided.

Meat, fish, poultry: All tender kinds are included, and may be baked, boiled, broiled, pan-broiled, or roasted.

Eggs may be prepared as desired.

Vegetables and fruit: Soft cooked vegetables and cooked, canned, or ripe fresh fruit are included. Strained vegetables are acceptable when combined with other foods as in a milk soup or a casserole with ground meat or baked with egg.

Vegetable and fruit juices are included if not strongly acid. In peptic disorders these products may be taken with other foods. When the bland diet is used in conditions where the mouth or throat is sore, highly acid foods are avoided. Orange juice with a pH ranging from 3.30 to 4.34 may still cause pain. The American Home Economics Association's *Handbook of Food Preparation,* 6th ed, (1971) lists the pH of some common foods.

Breads, cereals: Cooked or ready-to-eat whole grain or enriched breads and cereals are included. When symptoms are acute, finely-milled cereals and white bread are used. At all times products containing coarse fibers or large amounts of seeds, nuts, etc., are excluded.

Moderate amounts of fats, sweets, salt, flavorings, and seasonings are used.

Decaffeinated beverages are included.

Foods usually restricted in a bland diet are these:

Coarse-fibered, pickled, salted, smoke-salted, and highly seasoned meats and fish.

Highly concentrated soups and gravies made from soup bases.

Vegetables and fruit with coarse fibers, tough skins, and seeds.

Pickles and relishes, strongly acid foods and juices, acid-containing soft drinks, alcoholic beverages.

Very sweet or rich foods.

Nuts or other hard particles such as popcorn, seed spices.

Pepper, chili powder, cloves, and mustard. These have been found to be irritating to the gastric mucosa (Schneider et al, 1956).

Coffee, tea, or soft drinks that contain caffeine. According to Turner (1970, pages 44 and 45), "A cup of strong coffee contains about 0.1 to 0.15 gm of caffeine" and "A cup of strong tea prepared from one teaspoon dried leaves contains about 0.1 gm of caffeine". Caffeine, when consumed without food, may increase the acid output of the stomach.

The use of alcohol, drugs, and tobacco is at the discretion of the physician.

MODIFIED RESIDUE DIETS

The modified residue diets include (1) a low residue diet, and (2) a restricted shortened fiber diet.

The low residue diet aims to provide as little residue in the intestinal tract as possible. It may be used as a preparative diet for intestinal surgery, for certain X-ray diagnostic procedures, and at times after intestinal surgery. For patients who have undergone colostomy current practice in their dietary care is to progress from extreme limitation in residue to a soft diet and then to a general diet as soon as their condition permits.

Diet Plan: Low Residue Regimen

Foods are limited for a short time to these:

Tender cuts of meats, fish, poultry; crisp bacon

Eggs (not fried)

Clear, cooked fruit and vegetable juices

Enriched white bread, refined cereals, rice, pastas

Plain crackers, cookies, cakes

Butter, margarine; sugar, jellies

Broth, tea, coffee, decaffeinated beverages

Vegetables and fruit other than the juices as indicated above are not used. See "Flatulence," Appendix I for juice selection.

Milk and cream have no fiber, but do contribute to bulk, so they are generally excluded. In conditions such as Crohn's disease, such exclusion is unnecessary.

An alternative preparative nutrition program where minimum bowel residue is desired is the use of a low residue formula of conventional foods or a nutritionally adequate synthetic diet. One such synthetic product, Vivonex®, is presently available. Fluid intake must be watched when products of high ismolality are used to avoid general dehydration from the concentrated mixture and the hyperosmolarity of the blood. See section on liquid diets.

Diet Plan: Restricted Fiber Diet

A restricted fiber diet allows cooked fruits and vegetables, restricting only those which have long stringy fibers. It aims to provide hydrophyllic bulk and to omit food materials such as dried beans or soy products that may cause gas in the intestinal tract. It follows the pattern of the daily food guide but includes fruits and

vegetables with soft fiber, and shortens the fiber in stringy vegetables to avoid the possible formation of an entangled ball or the
pile-up of coarse materials in the intestine. This diet may include
reduced or increased amounts of soft fiber depending on the number and size of the servings of allowed vegetables and fruit in the
day's meals.

The soft diet is modified in fiber in that it excludes vegetables
and fruit with coarse structural fibers and tough skins, grain foods
that are not finely milled, and meats with firm connective tissue.
In some cases this degree of modification is sufficient.

Thorough mastication is recommended to breakup food materials for ease in digestion.

Since some disintegration of cellulose materials and pectic substances occurs during cooking, most vegetables should be thoroughly cooked. Skins and seeds should be removed. Long structural
fibers which may cause difficulty in their usual state are acceptable
if blenderized or chopped to reduce the length of the fibers and to
break up any particles. Lettuce and raw carrot, if shredded, and
tomatoes with seeds and skins removed may be used. Vegetables
usually excluded unless thoroughly blenderized are celery, collards,
kale, turnip greens, whole kernel corn. See "Flatulence,"
Appendix I.

Cooked, canned, or ripe fresh fruits may be used but seeds of
berries and tough skins are avoided. Fresh fruits with woody fibers
are avoided. As a general rule, foods with a fiber content of over
1.0 gram per serving portion are excluded. Total fiber consumed
during the day must be considered. Handbook 8, *Composition of
Foods Raw, Processed, Prepared* (Watt and Merrill, 1963) lists
the fiber content of foods.

Tender cuts of meat, or less tender cuts cooked slowly with moist
heat, are included. Long cooking converts the collagen in connective
tissue to gelatin.

Smooth peanut butter may be used.

Finely-milled whole grain or enriched breads and cereals are
included as well as pastas, white rice, and prepared cereals with a
minimum of bran. Breads with coarse bran in them such as cracked
wheat and pumpernickel are not used.

Nuts, popcorn, and seed spices are not included.

In prescribing diets and in selecting foods for inclusion, consideration must be given to the condition for which the diet is ordered. Narrowing of the intestinal lumen (Crohn's disease) does not require elimination of small seeds. Diverticulosis where the seeds might become physically entrapped requires their elimination. Research has been directed toward evaluating the efficacy of the traditional *low* fiber diet in treatment of intestinal conditions.

> In diverticulosis present clinical practice emphasizes foods that contribute to a soft bulky stool. Almy (1965) says, *"In the long term management (of diverticular disease of the colon) the traditional low residue foods should be exchanged for a high residue diet supplemented by hydrophyllic colloids as the presence of a larger fecal mass in the sigmoid may make impossible the close approximation of the walls and the development of high intraluminal pressures in very short segments."*

Burkitt et al (1972) suggested that dietary fiber has a role in the prevention of certain diseases of the large bowel. Hunt (1972) reviewed the changes in dietary treatment.

When diarrhea is present the diet will depend on the cause and duration of this symptom. Less than the usual amount of bulk in the diet does not usually appear to be beneficial. When diarrhea is severe and/or prolonged, replacement of fluid and electrolyte losses, particularly potassium, is important. Depending on the person's condition the soft or general diet may be used. In acute infections he may not be able to take anything but liquids. In the diarrheas of malabsorption syndromes therapy must be directed toward the primary cause. See the restricted gluten and the restricted lactose diets as examples. The potassium values of some common foods are given in Table VI-5, Section VI.

Fiber and Residue

Hardinge et al (1958) found that the average American diet contains from 8.4 to 12.2 grams of fiber per day whereas vegetarian diets range as high as 23.9 grams per day.

Restriction of the amount of fiber reduces the amount of residue in the bowel. According to Guyton (1971) "the feces normally are about three-fourths water and one-fourth solid matter composed of about 30% dead bacteria, 10 to 20% fat, 10 to 20% inorganic

TABLE IV-2
SUMMARY OF SOFT DIET MODIFICATIONS

	Soft Diet	Mechanical Soft Diet	Smooth (Pureed) Diet	Bland Diet	Low Residue Diet	Modified Residue Restricted Fiber Diet (Soft short fiber)
Milk Group						
Milk	2 cups	2 cups	2 cups	2 cups	None	2 cups
Cheeses	Cottage and plain cured	Cottage and plain cured	Cottage and plain cured	Cottage and plain cured	None	Cottage and plain cured
Meat Group						
Any tender meat, poultry or fish	4 to 6 exchanges. In pieces or serving cuts	Ground after cooking. Fish or soft meats need not be ground	Blenderized	See soft diet	Same as soft diet, but larger servings	See soft diet
Bacon	Crisp	See soft diet	Generally not tolerated	See soft diet	Same as soft diet but larger servings	See soft diet
Eggs—3 per week	Prepared in any manner	See soft diet	See soft diet	See soft diet	See soft diet	See soft diet
Peanut butter, smooth only	As desired within caloric limits	See soft diet	See soft diet	See soft diet	None	See soft diet
Vegetables and Fruits						
Well cooked vegetables, lettuce, shredded raw carrots and ripe tomatoes	4 to 5 servings. All without coarse fibers or tough skins	See soft diet. Any soft item	See soft diet. Strained or blenderized	See soft diet	None. Omit all but clear fruit or vegetable juices	See soft diet. High fiber fruits or vegetables must be cooked and blenderized to shorten fibers. Avoid tough skins and seeds.
Potatoes	See diet plans					
Cooked, canned, or fresh ripe fruit	Any kind except coarse fibered					
Fruit and vege-	Any kind	Any kind	Avoid acid	Omit strongly	Clear juices	Any juice or

			foods if throat or mouth lesions present	acid fruits and vegetables if mouth or throat lesions	only	nectar
...table juices						See soft diet
Bread—Cereal Group Enriched bread and cereals, Finely milled whole-grain breads and cereals; pastas, rice	As desired. At least 4 servings. Avoid cracked wheat	See soft diet. Provide liquid to soften	See soft diet. Tough crusts must be softened. No crisp foods	See soft diet	White bread. Refined cereals and pastas. White rice. No whole grain products	See soft diet
Fats and Oils	As desired within caloric needs	See soft diet	See soft diet	See soft diet	See soft diet	See soft diet
Sweets and Sugars	In limited amounts	See soft diet	See soft diet	Concentrated sweets are avoided	No milk or fruit desserts	See soft diet
Beverages Coffee and tea and alternates, Fruit-flavored drinks, Soft drinks	As desired	See soft diet	Avoid acid drinks including soft drinks if throat or mouth lesion is present	Avoid tea, coffee and alcohol unless allowed by physician. No soft drinks	Clear beverages only. Fruit-flavored drinks and soft drinks allowed	As desired
Soups	Any soups not highly seasoned or containing whole kernel corn	See soft diet	Same as soft diet, but blenderized	See soft diet	Avoid all except stock soups, with allowed cereal products only. No milk or vegetable soups	See soft diet
Seasonings	Avoid pickles, condiments, raw onions, garlic and peppers. Limit spices and herbs.	See soft diet	See soft diet	See soft diet. Also avoid mustard, chili, peppers and cloves.	Avoid all vegetables except clear juice. Avoid seed spices, pickles, condiments and relishes.	See soft diet. Also avoid seed spices

matter, 2 to 3% protein, and 30% undigested roughage of food and dried constituents of digestive juices such as bile pigments and sloughed epithelial cells."

The amount and quality of fiber in fruits and vegetables varies with the locality and season of its growth, age when picked, degree of preparation for cooking, and length of time and method of cooking.

In respect to residue other than fiber, foods may be listed in general in increasing order of residue production as follows: protein, fats, milk, digestible carbohydrates, and carbohydrates with indigestible material (Weinstein et al, 1961). Their report includes the following table and the references from which it was compiled. Note that the quantity of food taken in 24 hours was limited, with one exception, to a single kind.

Food Residue

Diet	Quantity taken (gm) per 24 hours	Net weight (gm) per 24 hours	Dry Weight (gm) per 24 hours
Mixed	. . .	100-150	20-30
Meat	1,435	64.0	17.2
White Bread	1,237	109.0	28.9
Dark Bread	1,360	815.0	115.8
Potato	3,078	635.0	93.8
Peas	960	927.1	124.0
Milk	3,075	174.0	40.6
Milk	3 quarts	114.5	25.3
Milk	1,680	. . .	21.5
Cabbage, raw	210	700 (approx.)	. . .

Milk is generally considered to possess moderate residue-producing effects. J. Watts et al (1963) studied the amounts of intestinal residue excreted following ingestion of a low residue diet plus various dairy foods. They found that solids excreted were highest during sweet milk feeding and lowest during periods when cheese or a combination of dairy foods (some combinations including sweet milk) were fed. Buttermilk produced less solids than sweet milk. Although the highest excretion of total ash occurred during sweet milk feeding, the lowest excretion of calcium in the feces occurred at this time.

TABLE IV-3a
CALCULATED NUTRIENT ESTIMATES OF
QUALITATIVE DIETS AS SERVED IN A HOSPITAL

Nutrients	Unit	Recommended Dietary Allowances Man 51+ Years	Recommended Dietary Allowances Woman 51+ Years	Hospital Full Liquid Diet	Hospital Smooth Diet
Food energy	Calorie	2,400	1,800	2,020	2,425
Protein	gm	56	46	90	115
Fat	gm	—	—	75	100
Carbohydrate	gm	—	—	250	265
Calcium	gm	0.8	0.8	2.5	2.5
Phosphorus	gm	0.8	0.8	2.1	2.3
Iron	mg	10.0	10.0	6.0	11.0
Magnesium	mg	350	300	325	359
Sodium	mg	—	—	3,002	2,774
Sodium mEq				131	121
Potassium	mg	—	—	3,897	4,710
Potassium mEq				100	121
Vitamin A	IU	5,000	4,000	4,538	11,948
Vitamin E		15 IU	12 IU	2.7 mg	3.3 mg
Ascorbic acid	mg	45.0	45.0	79.0	105.0
Folacin	mg	0.4	0.4	—	—
Niacin equivalent	mg	16.0	12.0	25.0	36.0
Riboflavin	mg	1.5	1.1	3.8	4.2
Thiamin	mg	1.2	1.0	1.0	1.2
Vitamin B$_6$	mg	2.0	2.0	1.3	1.8
Vitamin B$_{12}$	mcg	3.0	3.0	8.4	9.2

TABLE IV-3b
CALCULATED NUTRIENT ESTIMATES OF
QUALITATIVE DIETS AS SERVED IN A HOSPITAL

Nutrients	Unit	Hospital Mechanical Soft Diet	Hospital Bland Diet	Hospital Restricted Fiber Diet
Food energy	Calorie	2,131	2,305	2,200
Protein	gm	99	90	95
Fat	gm	83	100	95
Carbohydrate	gm	253	270	250
Calcium	gm	1.3	1.1	1.2
Phosphorus	gm	1.7	1.4	1.5
Iron	mg	14.8	14.0	14.0
Magnesium	mg	249	291	288
Sodium	mg	4,297	2,824	3,588
Sodium mEq		187	123	156
Potassium	mg	3,270	2,860	2,968
Potassium mEq		84	73	76
Vitamin A	IU	8,595	9,698	7,257
Vitamin E	mg	4.8	6.8	5.8
Ascorbic acid	mg	87.0	69.0	90.0
Folacin		—	—	—
Niacin equivalent	mg	27.7	31.0	31.0
Riboflavin	mg	2.7	2.1	2.2
Thiamin	mg	1.7	1.3	1.4
Vitamin B$_6$	mg	1.6	1.7	1.8
Vitamin B$_{12}$	mcg	4.6	4.5	5.8

DIET FOLLOWING GASTRIC SURGERY—
DUMPING SYNDROME

The dumping syndrome may occur following ingestion of food in a person who has undergone gastric surgery. The normal processes of digestion and absorption are altered by the surgery, the extent of which will influence the degree of impairment. Dietary care is directed toward the prevention of this syndrome.

1. When there is loss of the holding capacity of the stomach, it can no longer serve as a reservoir for food, releasing small amounts of chyme at a time.

2. There is reduction of the gastric secretions including the intrinsic factor required for B_{12} absorption, and there may be reduction of the digestive secretions of the intestine, pancreas, and gall-bladder.

3. Motility is impaired, and the mixing of food with digestive secretions in the stomach and intestine may be incomplete.

4. Absorption is reduced. The reduction of gastric secretions and inadequate mixing will influence absorption in the small intestine.

5. Following ingestion, food may be dumped precipitously into the jejunum causing a rapid change in the osmotic relationships of the intestinal tract. A shift of the intravascular fluid occurs to dilute the hyperosmotic content of the jejunum. The plasma volume begins to fall within 10 minutes, and the symptoms of nausea, fullness, sweating, and faintness follow (Davenport, 1968, page 180). The objectives of the diet are:

1. To adjust the day's food to the reduced storage capacity of the stomach.
2. To select the kind and modify the form of foods to the lessened mechanical action and to reduce digestive secretions.
3. To eliminate those foods (mono- and disaccharides) that contribute to a hypertonic solution; and to limit all carbohydrates.
4. To limit the amount of fluid ingested with a meal.
5. To promote slow eating and thorough chewing of foods.
6. To emphasize the B vitamins, especially B_6, B_{12}, and folic acid. These are poorly absorbed under conditions resulting from gastrectomy. Mineral and vitamin supplements are recommended.

Diet Plan for Dumping Syndrome

The diet is moderate in protein, increased in fat, and low in carbohydrate. Small amounts of food should be offered at one time and frequent feedings planned throughout the day. At least six meals are provided.

When foods are offered, at first they should be somewhat bland, low in liquid content and fiber, and moderate in temperature. They should require some chewing and should be eaten slowly. If a dry meal is required fluids should not be offered with food or for 30 to 45 minutes preceding or following a meal. When fluids are permitted with a meal the quantity should not exceed 4 ounces (1/2 cup) initially.

The diet must meet the needs presented by the individual patient. It is accepted better if it includes foods that are familiar and well-liked. There may be loss of appetite. Also, the experience of the dumping syndrome may lead to a disinclination to eat.

Frequent monitoring following surgery is essential, and a careful approach to the planning of feedings is important. Since absorption is impaired, foods of high nutritive value low in osmotic concentration should be emphasized.

If symptoms occur when a patient is taking a meal in a seated position there may be less difficulty if he eats while reclining. He should lie down after eating. If nausea develops the feeding should be stopped, and food should not be offered again until the next meal period. Some of any of the foods in the diet outline may be used but in lesser quantities until symptoms subside.

As tolerance increases the diet may be liberalized. The quantities of foods at a meal and the kinds selected should be altered gradually so that a more normal eating pattern will be resumed. A maintenance diet is a modified fiber diet, moderate in protein, high in fat, and low in carbohydrate with restriction of mono- and disaccharides, with return to regular foods as tolerated.

Two diet outlines are included: a beginning diet of about 1200 calories, and a maintenance diet of about 2000. If weight gain is desirable, additions in meats, potatoes, and refined cereals may be made. Usually the first foods included in the meals following surgery are:

1. Tender meats, chicken, liver, crisp bacon; soft or hard-cooked eggs; canned, fresh, or frozen fish; cottage and cream cheese; smooth peanut butter. Meats and other protein foods baked, broiled, boiled, or poached with a minimum of fat are used instead of fried foods.

2. Soups, when used, should be counted toward the fluid allowance.
3. Vegetables and fruits should be somewhat low in fiber and well-cooked. Fruit and vegetable juices may be gelled to slow down their intake. Purees may be required for a short time, but soft, well-cooked vegetables and ripe fruit should be offered soon.
   Avoid vegetables and fruit with coarse fibers, and tough skins.
4. Well-cooked or ready-to-eat refined cereals, pastas, rice, white potatoes, enriched bread, toast, melba toast, soda crackers, zwiebach, breadsticks (plain) are useful because they require chewing.
   Do not use sugar-coated cereals, sweetened or highly seasoned crackers.
5. Butter, margarine, salad dressings that are not strong in seasoning and acid.
6. Sugar is not included in the beginning diet, and until tolerance is established, it is customary to avoid ice cream, ice milk, sherbet, sweetened puddings, cookies, cakes with or without frosting, sweetened beverages, jams, jellies, honey, molasses, syrups, candies.
7. Milk is not included in the beginning diet because some patients

TABLE IV-4
MAINTENANCE DIET FOLLOWING GASTRIC SURGERY

Food Group: *1200 Calories*	Amount	Protein	Fat	Carbohydrate	Calories
Milk:	2 cups	16	20	24	340
Vegetables: List 2A, page 16	1 exch	—	—	— Negligible — — —	
List 2B, page 17	1 exch	2	0	7	35
White potato	1 exch	2	0	15	70
Fruit, unsweetened:	1 exch	0	0	20	80
Bread—cereals:	3 exch	6	0	45	210
Meat, fish, poultry, eggs:	5 exch	35	25	0	375
Butter, margarine:	3 exch	0	15	0	135
Totals and percentage calorie		61	60	111	1245
distribution:		(20%)	(44%)	(36%)	
Food Group: *2000 Calories*					
Milk:	2 cups	16	20	24	340
Cream, 20%:	¼ cup	2	12	3	125
Vegetables: List 2A, page 16	1 exch	—	—	— Negligible — — —	
List 2B, page 17	2 exch	4	0	14	70
White potato	1 exch	2	0	15	70
Fruit and fruit juices, unsweetened:	4 exch	0	0	40	160
Bread—cereals:	6 exch	12	0	90	420
Meat, fish, poultry, eggs:	8 exch	56	40	0	600
Butter, margarine, mild salad dressings:	6 exch	0	30	0	270
Totals and percentage calorie		92	102	186	2055
distribution:		(18%)	(45%)	(37%)	

Start with small quantities of cooked fruits and vegetables. Add coarse-fibered vegetables with care, small amounts only. Lettuce is generally well-tolerated.
Add raw fruit in small amounts until good tolerance is demonstrated.

experience milk intolerance following gastric surgery (Spencer and Welbourn, 1968). When introduced the quantity should be 2 to 3 ounces at a time and offered between meals. Milk may also then be included in a meal when combined with other foods as in a thick soup, a vegetable puree, or a vegetable custard. If milk intolerance is suspected the physician may prescribe a lactose-free or a low lactose diet.

8. Foods that are high in seasoning or salt or that are strongly acid are not included until tolerance has been established, and then should be used only in moderation. The basic pattern of the soft diet may be the beginning point for modification according to the extent of the surgery and the patient's desires.

9. If and when some sugar is included it should be used in combination with other foods as in a custard, cornstarch puddings, or mildly sweetened fruit sauce. The total amount of sugar should be spread throughout the day.

POST-CARDIAC SURGERY DIETARY REGIMEN*

Rationale

The object of the diet is to provide foods that are easy to handle, to chew, and to digest.

Beverages containing substantial amounts of caffeine are not used.

Sodium may need to be restricted; if so, the level will be prescribed.

Boullion which is high in salt is not included.

Cholesterol is limited, as a routine, to under 300 mg per day.

Fluids must frequently be limited; the degree of restriction varies and depends on the status of the individual.

Diet Plan

The diet progresses from liquid to the soft diet with daily additions to a maintenance diet; and the following outline may be used for children or adults by adjusting the portion sizes to the needs of the individual.

Liquids that are served to the limit of the fluid restrictions are these:

Water

Soft drinks such as gingerale and 7-Up®

*Consultants: Miss Rochelle Schmitz, RN, Head Nurse, Cardio-Vascular Surgery, University of Wisconsin Center for Health Sciences; William P. Young, MD, Professor of Surgery, University of Wisconsin Medical School

Apple, grape, pineapple juice or fruit nectars, all enriched with ascorbic acid. Clear fruit-flavored drinks may be used. Orange juice is avoided because the oil present may be irritating. Clear gels may be made with the allowed fruit juices and nectars. They would be counted as part of the fluid intake. Most young patients express a preference for fruit-flavored drinks.

Weak tea, either hot or iced

Solid foods may usually be offered after one day on liquids only, but progression is determined on an individual basis as soon as the patient can tolerate food. Usually a maintenance diet is suitable on the fifth day postoperative.

Cardiac Surgical Soft Diet
Suggested Plan for Addition of Solid Foods

Breakfast, 1st day postoperative	Additions on days indicated
Fruit juice	4th day: egg prepared in any manner
Cereal, cooked or ready-to-eat	
Milk; skim for weight-watchers or patients with coronary disease.	
Toast with spread	
Luncheon or Supper	
Soup as allowed on Bland Diet	2nd day: simple dessert
Toast with spread	3rd day: canned fruit without seeds or skin may be substituted for simple dessert.
Milk	
Dinner	
Soup (see above) or small serving tender meat or fish or cottage cheese	2nd day: same as first day, or a smooth ground meat or fish sandwich with mayonnaise may replace the serving of meat or fish.
Simple dessert: choose one (1) smooth plain pudding, ice cream, or sherbet (no nuts, fruit chunks) plain sugar cooky angel cake	3rd day: a serving of mashed or baked potato, or substitute a plain casserole for serving

Milk

of meat or fish.
4th day: a soft vegetable
as included in the
Bland Diet.

Spreads for toast will depend on the patient's preference. Clear jellies, smooth peanut butter, margarine, butter, or cream cheese are satisfactory unless the butter or cream cheese must be limited by cholesterol restriction.

Sandwich suggestion: With fluid restriction patients generally find the smooth, mayonnaise-moistened salad-type (no celery, pickles, or nuts) sandwich more easily eaten. Other sandwiches include sliced chicken or turkey with mayonnaise, peanut butter with jelly. "Finger" sandwiches are easily handled.

Egg yolks are limited to two per week to control cholesterol intake.

If salt is further restricted, see the controlled sodium diets.

REFERENCES

Modifications in Consistency of Food

Almy, TP: Divertical disease of the colon; the new look. *Gastroenterol, 49*: 109, 1965.

American Dietetic Association: Position paper on bland diet in treatment of chronic duodenal ulcer. *J Am Dietet A, 59*:244, 1971.

Bayless, TM (Guest ed.): Symposium: Structure and function of the gut. *Am J Clin Nutr, 24*:43, 1971.

Buchman, E, et al: Unrestricted diet in the treatment of duodenal ulcer. *Gastroenterol, 56*:1016, 1969.

Burkitt, DP, et al: Effect of dietary fiber on stool and transit times, and its role in the causation of disease. *Lancet, II*:1408, 1972.

French, AB; Cook, BB; Pollard, HM: Nutritional problems after gastro-intestinal surgery. *Med Clin North Am, 53*:1389, 1969.

Gardner, FH: Nutritional management of chronic diarrhea in adults. *JAMA, 180*:147, 1962.

Guyton, AC: *Textbook of Medical Physiology,* 4th ed. Philadelphia, Saunders, 1971, Part 9.

Hunt, T: Digestive diseases: The changing scene. *Br Med J, 4*:689, 1972.

Ingelfinger, FJ: Regional absorption. *Am J Surg, 114*:388, 1967.

————: Gastrointestinal absorption. *Nutr Today, 2*:2, Mar, 1967.

————: The dietotherapy of gastrointestinal complaints. *Viewpoints on Dig Diseases, 1* (no 3):1, 1969. (This is a leaflet published 5 times yearly by American Gastroenterological Association and Digestive Foundation, Dept of Medicine, Chapel Hill, North Carolina.)

Joint Committee, American Dietetic Association and American Medical Association: Diet as related to gastrointestinal function. *JAMA, 176*:935, 1961.

Lennard-Jones, JE: Is diet a treatment for peptic ulcer? A review of the evidence. *Rendic R Gastroenterol, 2*:189, 1970.

Parks, TG: Divertical disease of the colon. *Postgrad Med J, 44*:680, 1968.

Schneider, MA; De Luca, V; Grey, SJ: The effect of spice ingestion upon the stomach. *Am J Gastroenterology, 26*:722, 1956.

Shils, ME: Nutritional problems arising from the treatment of cancer. *CA, 20*:188, 1970.

Solomon, B: Preliminary report on the dietary management of patients with advanced carcinoma. *Md Med J, 18*:77, May, 1969.

Spiro, H: *Clinical Gastroenterology.* New York, Macmillan, 1970.

Truelove, WI; Reynell, PC: *Diseases of Digestive System,* 2nd ed. London, Blackwell, 1972.

Winawer, SJ; Zamcheck, N: Pathophysiology of small intestine resection in man. *Progress in Gastroenterology, 1*:339, 1968.

Zegarelli, EV, et al: Maintaining the oral and general health of the oral cancer patient, Part Two. *CA, 19*:232, 1969.

Modified Fiber, Residue and pH of Foods

American Home Economics Association: *Handbook of Food Preparation,* 6th ed. Washington, DC, American Home Economics Association, 1971.

Cummings, JH: Dietary fibre. *Gut, 14*:69, 1973.

Hardinge, MG; Chambers, AC; Crooks, H; Stare, FJ: Nutritional studies of vegetarians, Part three: Dietary levels of fiber. *Am J Clin Nutr, 6*:523, 1958.

————; Swarner, JB; Crooks, H: Carbohydrates in foods. *J Am Diet Assoc, 46*:197, 1965.

Watts, JH, et al: Fecal solids excreted by young men following the ingestion of dairy foods. *Am J Dig Dis, 8*:364, 1963.

Diet Following Gastric Surgery

Abott, WE; Krieger, H; Levey, S; Bradshaw, J: The etiology and management of the dumping syndrome following a gastroenterostomy or subtotal gastrectomy. *Gastroenterol, 39*:12, 1960.

Bolt, RJ: Gastric evacuation and clinical syndromes. *Med Clin North Am, 53*:1403, 1969.

Buchwald, H: The dumping syndrome and its treatment. A review and presentation of cases. *Am J Surg, 116*:81, 1968.

Davenport, HD: *Physiology of the Digestive Tract,* 2nd ed. Chicago, Year Book Med Publishers, Inc, 1966.

Pittman, AC; Robinson, FW: Dumping syndrome: Control by diet. *J Am Diet Assoc, 34*:596, 1958.

Silver, D; Porter, JM; Acinapura, AJ; McGregor, FH: The pathogenesis and management of the dumping syndrome. *Surg Sci, 3*:365, 1966.

Sjoberg, HE: Nutritional studies on dumping syndrome. 3, Retention of orally administered calcium in patients after gastrectomy. *Am J Dig Dis, 12*:1156, 1967.

Spencer, J; Welbourn, RB: Milk intolerance following gastric operations with special reference to lactase deficiency. *Brit J Surg, 55*:261, 1968.

SECTION V

MODIFICATIONS IN CALORIES

DIETS WITH INCREASED CALORIES:
3,000 AND 3,500 CALORIES

DIETS WITH INCREASED CALORIES are frequently used for the person with increased metabolic need and for the person in a depleted nutritional state. Poor food habits, chronic illness with concomitant loss of appetite, poor absorption, increased nutrient loss all contribute to a state of nutrient depletion. Alcoholics are frequently malnourished.

Under all circumstances dietary treatment is directed to the condition present in the individual. Appetite will dictate the regimen used.

Diet Plan

These diets provide calories, protein, minerals, and vitamins well above the average levels. The caloric value of these diets will fluctuate from day to day; therefore they are not suitable for anyone whose intake must be constant.

A gradual approach to increasing calories is desirable. Soft foods that require little chewing encourage eating. Interval feedings, if used, should contribute to the day's desired intake. Sweetened beverages or desserts between meals tend to blunt the appetite for the next meal.

In the hospital the General Diet is used as the basis for high caloric plans. Substantial between-meal feedings are included in the daily routine. No unusual foods, or foods requiring purchase of special ingredients are used. At times the person who needs to eat a lot of food tires before the meal is consumed. An effort is made to provide foods that are easy to eat and that do not require much chewing.

90

TABLE V-1

QUANTITIES OF FOOD AND CALORIE AND PROTEIN VALUES
DIETS WITH INCREASED CALORIES

Food Group	Amount for 3,000 Calories	Calories	Protein	Amount for 3,500 Calories	Calories	Protein
Milk group						
Milk, whole	4 cups	680	32	4 cups	680	32
Cream, light	1/3 cup	120	3	1/3 cup	120	3
Meat group	6 exchanges	450	42	8 exchanges	600	56
Vegetables						
List A	As desired	Negligible		As desired	Negligible	
List B	3 exchanges	105	6	3 exchanges	105	6
Fruit	3 exchanges	120	0	3 exchanges	120	0
Bread-cereals	6 exchanges	420	12	9 exchanges	630	18
Fats and oils	7 exchanges	315	0	9 exchanges	405	0
Sugar	4 teaspoons	80	0	4 teaspoons	80	0
High calorie food	2 servings	700	6	2 servings	700	6
	Totals	2990	101		3440	121

TABLE V-2

CALCULATED NUTRIENT ESTIMATES OF DIETS WITH
INCREASED CALORIES AS SERVED IN A HOSPITAL

Nutrients	Unit	Recommended Dietary Allowances Man 51+ Years	Recommended Dietary Allowances Woman 51+ Years	Hospital 3,000 Calorie Diet	Hospital 3,500 Calorie Diet
Food energy	Calorie	2,400	1,800	3,035	3,505
Protein	gm	56	46	120	140
Fat	gm	—	—	—	—
Carbohydrate	gm	—	—	355	385
Calcium	gm	0.8	0.8	1.8	2.0
Phosphorus	gm	0.8	0.8	2.1	2.4
Iron	mg	10.0	10.0	17.0	20.0
Magnesium	mg	350	300	393	423
Sodium	mg	—	—	4,643	5,539
Sodium mEq				202	241
Potassium	mg	—	—	4,064	4,303
Potassium mEq				104	110
Vitamin A	IU	5,000	4,000	8,338	9,393
Vitamin E		15 IU	12 IU	8.4 mg	10.7 mg
Ascorbic acid	mg	45.0	45.0	110.0	110.0
Folacin	mg	0.4	0.4	—	—
Niacin	mg	16.0	12.0	36.0	41.0
Riboflavin	mg	1.5	1.1	3.2	3.6
Thiamin	mg	1.2	1.0	1.8	2.2
Vitamin B_6	mg	2.0	2.0	2.1	2.3
Vitamin B_{12}	mcg	3.0	3.0	6.5	7.4

The diet outlines presented here (Table V-1) specify minimum amounts of food to provide 3,000 and 3,500 calories, respectively. Since no maximum limits are set, it would be possible for the caloric level to be higher. The protein and calorie values used in these calculations are the rounded averages of the standard food exchange lists. A high caloric food has been indicated in the diet plans to include an average value for a special entrée, a favorite dessert, or a milkshake. One serving is counted as 350 calories. A spread such as peanut butter is a concentrated food and may be used, when appropriate, to add its nutritional value to the diet. Jelly may be substituted for one or more of the servings of sugar at the rate of 20 calories per teaspoon.

CONVENTIONAL DIETS WITH DECREASED CALORIES (3 MEALS PER DAY)

Low calorie diets are intended to create a negative balance resulting in weight loss. To serve as a rough guide a diet with a deficit of 500 calories needed to maintain body weight should produce a weight loss of about one pound a week.

Diet Plans

Two plans for use in weight reduction are outlined in this section. Either should be individualized to suit a person's requirements for nutrition, his likes and dislikes of foods, his daily routine, and his economic status. In planning these diets care should be taken to select whole grain breads and cereals in the quantities allowed; to include frequently lean pork for its thiamin value, and green leafy vegetables for their contributions in minerals and vitamins; and to provide daily a good source of vitamin C. At least one of the servings of fat should be a good source of vitamin E such as a vegetable oil or margarine. Skim milk should be fortified in vitamins A and D.

Weight Reduction Diets: Standard Protein, Reduced Fat, and Moderately Reduced Carbohydrate

The conventional weight reduction diets are suitable for most persons. They conform to distribution of calories like these:

Calories	Protein	Fat	Carbohydrate
1,000	27%	28%	45%
1,200	27%	30%	43%
1,500	23%	30%	47%

The protein, fat, carbohydrate, and calorie values used in planning the conventional weight reduction diets are the rounded averages of the standard food exchanges. The amounts of food and the protein, fat, carbohydrate and caloric values for one 1,000 calorie diet, two 1,200 calorie diets, and two 1,500 calorie diets are outlined here (Tables V-3, 4 and 5).

TABLE V-3

CONVENTIONAL 1000 CALORIE DIET

This 1000 calorie diet is suitable for adult use. Note that the estimates for magnesium and vitamin B₆ are lower than the recommended dietary allowances for those nutrients for the man and woman 23 to 50 years of age; and low in iron for the woman also.

Food Group	Size of Exchange	Number of Exchanges	Protein gm	Fat gm	Carbohydrate gm	Calories
Milk, skim	8 ounce cup	2 exchanges	16	—	24	160
Vegetables						
List A, page 16	Not fixed	As desired	— — — — Negligible — — — —			
List B, page 17	½ cup	2 exchanges	4	0	14	70
Fruit	See list	3 exchanges	0	0	30	120
Bread-cereals	See list	3 exchanges	6	0	45	210
Lean meat	1 ounce meat	5 exchanges	40	15	0	300
Egg	8/lb.	3 in week	3	2	0	34
Fats and oils	1 teaspoon	3 exchanges	0	15	0	135
		Totals	69	32	113	1029

TABLE V-4

CONVENTIONAL 1200 CALORIE DIET NUMBER I AND DIET NUMBER II

The 1200 calorie diet number I follows the pattern of the 1000 calorie diet. The 1200 calorie diet number II is suggested for those who pack a lunch or eat in a restaurant because it provides more bread and fat and less meat than the number I diet. These diets are also low in magnesium and vitamin B₆ in comparison with the recommended dietary allowances for the man and woman 23 to 50 years old, and low in iron for the woman. These diets are suitable only for adult use because the quantity of milk is insufficient for adolescents.

Food Group	Diet I					Diet II				
	Amount	Protein gm	Fat gm	Carbohydrate gm	Calories	Amount	Protein gm	Fat gm	Carbohydrate gm	Calories
Milk, skim	2 cups	16	—	24	160	2 cups	16	—	24	160
Vegetables										
List A	Not fixed	—	—	Negligible	—	Not fixed	—	—	Negligible	—
List B	2 exchanges	4	0	14	70	2 exchanges	4	0	14	70
Fruit	3 exchanges	0	0	30	120	3 exchanges	0	0	30	120
Bread-cereals	4 exchanges	8	0	60	280	5 exchanges	10	0	75	350
Lean meat	6 exchanges	48	18	0	360	5 exchanges	40	15	0	300
Egg	3 in week	3	2	0	34	3 in week	3	2	0	34
Fats and oils	4 exchanges	0	20	0	180	4 exchanges	0	20	0	180
Totals		79	40	128	1204		73	37	143	1214

TABLE V-5

CONVENTIONAL 1500 CALORIE DIET NUMBER I AND DIET NUMBER II

The 1500 calorie diet number I is planned for adults; the 1500 calorie diet number II for adolescents as well as adults. The greater amount of milk (4 cups instead of 2) provides for a greater dietary allowance of calcium.

The number I, 1500 calorie diet is low in magnesium for the 23 to 50 year old man; in iron and magnesium for the 23 to 50 year old woman. The number II, 1500 calorie diet is low in iron for boys and girls 15 to 18 years old, and in magnesium for boys.

Water adds to the total intake of magnesium. In communities with potable water at the level of 4.5 mg/100 gm (as in Madison, Wisconsin) 8 cups of water will bring all of these diets to the levels of the recommended dietary allowances for this nutrient.

| | Diet I | | | | | Diet II | | | | |
Food Group	Amount	Protein gm	Fat gm	Carbohydrate gm	Calories	Amount	Protein gm	Fat gm	Carbohydrate gm	Calories
Milk, skim	1 cup	8	—	12	80	4 cups	32	—	48	320
Milk, whole	1 cup	8	10	12	170	—	—	—	—	—
Vegetables										
List 2A, page 16	Not fixed	—	— Negligible —	—	—	Not fixed	—	— Negligible —	—	—
List 2B, page 17	3 exchanges	6	0	21	105	2 exchanges	4	0	14	70
Fruit	4 exchanges	0	0	40	160	2 exchanges	0	0	20	80
Bread-cereals	6 exchanges	12	0	90	420	6 exchanges	12	0	90	420
Lean meat	6 exchanges	48	18	0	360	6 exchanges	48	18	0	360
Egg	3 in week	3	2	0	34	3 in week	3	2	0	34
Fats and oils	4 exchanges	0	20	0	180	5 exchanges	0	25	0	225
Totals		85	50	175	1509		99	45	172	1509

TABLE V-6

CALCULATED NUTRIENT ESTIMATES OF CONVENTIONAL DIETS WITH
DECREASED CALORIES AS SERVED IN A HOSPITAL

Nutrients	Unit	1,000 Calorie	1,200 Calorie Number I	1,200 Calorie Number II Packed Lunch	1,500 Calorie Number I	1,500 Calorie Number II Packed Lunch
Food energy	Calorie	1,029	1,204	1,214	1,509	1,509
Protein	gm	69	79	73	85	99
Fat	gm	32	40	37	50	45
Carbohydrate	gm	113	128	143	175	172
Calcium	gm	1.0	1.0	1.0	1.1	1.7
Phosphorus	gm	1.2	1.3	1.2	1.4	1.8
Iron	mg	11.0	12.0	13.0	14.0	13.0
Magnesium	mg	213	222	226	273	316
Sodium	mg	3,026	3,175	3,193	3,742	3,706
Sodium mEq		132	138	139	163	161
Potassium	mg	2,728	2,960	2,900	3,369	3,693
Potassium mEq		70	76	74	86	95
Vitamin A	IU	5,363	5,784	5,936	6,336	7,062
Vitamin E	mg	3.1	3.4	3.6	4.1	3.7
Ascorbic acid	mg	87.0	89.0	89.0	101.0	94.0
Folacin	— — — — —	No calculation made			— — — — —	
Niacin equivalent	mg	25.0	28.0	26.0	32.0	32.0
Riboflavin	mg	2.0	2.9	2.1	2.3	3.1
Thiamin	mg	1.6	1.6	1.6	1.9	2.0
Vitamin B$_6$	mg	1.6	1.8	1.7	2.1	1.9
Vitamin B$_{12}$	mcg	5.2	5.4	5.2	5.8	7.3

DECREASED CALORIES: MULTI-MEAL
(6 MEALS PER DAY)

A low calorie multi-meal regimen for weight reduction developed by Gordon, Goldberg, and Chosy (1963) uses these caloric distributions:

Diet	Calories	Protein	Fat	Carbohydrate
A	1200	30-35%	42-47%	18-23%
B	1000	35-40%	40-45%	18-23%
C	1000	30-35%	38-43%	25-30%

These diets are intended especially for overweight individuals who fail to lose weight despite adherence to traditional reduction diets. However, they may be used for anyone who is overweight.

Plan A is suggested for use of most patients. If weight loss fails to occur with Plan A, Plan B may be effective. It is essentially the same as Plan A but has fewer calories. For those people who are unable to tolerate or accept the very low carbohydrate levels of Plans A and B, Plan C may be used. This contains more carbohydrate.

These diets are suitable for adult use. Modification would be necessary for adolescents in order to meet the recommended allowances for calcium, riboflavin, and ascorbic acid.

The nutritive values used in planning these diets are the conventional ones of the standard food exchanges, with one exception. Because the pattern is high in protein and restricted in fat the wide selection of the Meat Group Exchange List is not possible. Instead, the selection of protein foods is limited to those low in fat, and the

TABLE V-7
FOOD PLANS FOR MULTI-MEAL DECREASED CALORIE DIET

Food Group	Amount	Protein gm	Fat gm	Carbo- hydrate gm	Calories
Plan A, 1,200 Calories					
Milk, skim	2 cups	16	—	24	160
Vegetables					
List A	2 to 4 cups	— — — — Negligible — — — —			
List B	1 exchange	2	0	7	35
Fruit	2 exchanges	0	0	20	80
Bread-cereals	1 exchange	2	0	15	70
Lean meat, fish, poultry					
Cooked weight	10 exchanges	80	30	0	600
Egg (or lean meat exchange)	One	6	6	0	80
Fats and oils	4 teaspoons	0	20	0	180
		106	56	66	1,205
Plan B, 1,000 Calories					
Milk, skim	2 cups	16	—	24	160
Vegetables					
List A	2 to 4 cups	— — — — Negligible — — — —			
List B	1 exchange	2	0	7	35
Fruit	1 exchange	0	0	10	40
Bread-cereals	½ exchange	1	0	7	35
Lean meat, fish, poultry	10 exchanges	80	30	0	600
Egg (or lean meat exchange)	One	6	6	0	80
Fats and oils	2 teaspoons	0	10	0	90
		105	46	48	1,040
Plan C, 1,000 Calories					
Milk, skim	2 cups	16	—	24	160
Vegetables					
List A	2 to 4 cups	— — — — Negligible — — — —			
List B	1 exchange	2	0	7	35
Fruit	2 exchanges	0	0	20	80
Bread-cereals	1½ exchanges	3	0	22	105
Lean meat, fish, poultry	8 exchanges	64	24	0	480
Egg (or lean meat exchange)	One	6	6	0	80
Fats and oils	3 teaspoons	0	15	0	135
		91	45	73	1,075

TABLE V-8

CALCULATED NUTRIENT ESTIMATES OF MULTI-MEAL DECREASED CALORIE DIETS: HIGH PROTEIN, MODERATE FAT, AND GREATLY REDUCED CARBOHYDRATE

| | | Recommended Dietary Allowances | | Diets as Served in a Hospital | | |
| | | Man | Woman | Plan A | Plan B | Plan C |
Nutrients	*Unit*	*23-50 Years Old*	*23-50 Years Old*	*1,200 Calorie*	*1,000 Calorie*	*1,000 Calorie*
Food energy	Calorie	2,700	2,000	1,280	1,130	1,190
Protein	gm	56	46	120	105	98
Fat	gm	—	—	60	50	55
Carbohydrate	gm	—	—	65	65	80
Calcium	gm	0.8	0.8	1.0	1.0	1.0
Phosphorus	gm	0.8	0.8	1.6	1.5	1.4
Iron	mg	10.0	18.0	13.0	12.0	11.0
Magnesium	mg	350	300	247	230	217
Sodium	mg	—	—	2,689	2,481	2,721
Sodium mEq				117	108	118
Potassium	mg	—	—	2,970	2,738	2,653
Potassium mEq				76	70	68
Vitamin A	IU	5,000	4,000	7,002	6,993	7,149
Vitamin E	IU	15 IU	12 IU	8.0 mg	6.1 mg	7.5 mg
Ascorbic acid	mg	45.0	45.0	132.0	131.0	123.0
Folacin	mg	0.4	0.4	—	—	—
Niacin equivalent	mg	18.0	13.0	42.0	34.0	32.3
Riboflavin	mg	1.6	1.2	2.2	2.0	2.0
Thiamin	mg	1.4	1.0	1.4	1.2	1.2
Vitamin B_6	mg	2.0	2.0	2.0	1.7	1.6
Vitamin B_{12}	mcg	3.0	3.0	6.8	5.9	6.0

values for one exchange of any of these are 8 grams protein, 3 grams fat, and 60 calories. See Lean Meat Exchange List in Section One, Food Exchange System, page 23.

Diet Plans

A 48-hour fast is recommended to precede use of the diet to break the metabolic pattern of lipogenesis. During this period, coffee, tea, water, and low calorie beverages may be taken by the persons as much as desired. One cup of prepared dietetic gelatin may also be included daily.

Three plans have been formulated according to this regimen and are outlined in Table V-7. Important factors in planning these diets are:

1. The distribution of food throughout the day includes breakfast, dinner, lunch or supper, and three interval feedings or meals.

2. Protein foods of high biological value (of high replacement value from animal sources) are emphasized in this diet and included in *each* of the six meals for their high satiety value. Lean meat items only are selected; they are trimmed of separable fat before cooking, and are cooked without added fat unless the amount used is taken from the day's allowance. If trimmed of visible internal fat after cooking the fat value as eaten may be even lower than that listed for a *lean meat* exchange. Lean pork, fresh and cured, is an exceptional source of thiamin and should be included frequently.

3. At least part of the allowed fats in these diets should come from vegetable oils or margarines to ensure provision of essential fatty acids and vitamin E.

4. Carbohydrate foods include vegetables and fruits of low caloric value, and small amounts of grain products or alternates. Breads and cereals should be whole grain or enriched.

REFERENCES

Bortz, WM: Metabolic consequences of obesity. *Ann Intern Med, 71*:833, 1969.
Brodoff, BN (Conference Chairman): Adipose tissue metabolism and obesity. *Ann NY Acad Sci, 131*:1-683, 1965.
Cohn, C; Joseph, J: Effects of caloric intake and feeding frequency on carbohydrate metabolism of the rat. *J Nutr, 100*:78, 1970.

Fabry, P: *Feeding Patterns and Nutritional Adaptations.* Toronto, Butterworth, 1969.

————; Tepperman, J: Meal frequency: A possible factor in human pathology. *Am J Clin Nutr, 23*:1059, 1970.

Galton, DJ: *The Human Adipose Cell: A Model for Errors in Metabolic Regulation.* New York, Appleton-Century-Crofts, 1971.

Gordon, ES: Efficiency of energy metabolism in obesity. *Am J Clin Nutr, 21*:1480, 1968.

————: Obesity: Gluttony or genes? *Postgrad Med, 45*:95, 1969.

————: Metabolic aspects of obesity. *Adv Metab Discord, 4*:449, 1970.

————; Goldberg, M; Chosy, GJ: A new concept in the treatment of obesity. *JAMA, 186*:50, 1963.

Leveille, GA: Lipogenic adaptations related to pattern of food intake. *Nutr Rev, 30*:151, 1972.

Mayer, J: *Overweight: Causes, Cost and Control.* Englewood Cliffs, Prentice Hall, 1968.

Miller, AT, Jr: *Energy Metabolism.* Philadelphia, Davis, 1968.

Muiruri, KL; Leveille, GA: Metabolic adaptations in meal-fed rats: Effects of increased meal frequency or ad libitum feeding in rats previously adapted to a single daily meal. *J Nutr, 100*:450, 1970.

Renold, AE; Cahill, GF, Jr (Section Eds.): Adipose tissue. In Section V, *Handbook of Physiology.* Washington, DC, Amer Physiological Society, 1965.

Stirling, JL; Stock, MJ: Metabolic origins of thermogenesis induced by diet. *Nature, 220*:801, 1968.

Tepperman, J: *Metabolic and Endocrine Physiology,* 2nd ed. Chicago, Year Book Medical Publishers, 1968, Chaps 10, 12.

Wadhwa, PS, et al: Metabolic consequences of feeding frequency in man. *Am. J Clin Nutr, 26*:823, 1973.

University Hospitals, Dietary Dept: *Wisconsin Comprehensive Multimeal Weight Reduction Plans.* Madison, Univ of Wisconsin Medical Center.

Cellularity

Hirsch, J; Han, PH: Cellularity of rat adipose tissue: Effects of growth, starvation and obesity. *J Lipid Res, 10*:77, 1969.

Knittle, JL; Hirsch, J: Infantile nutrition as a determinant of adult adipose tissue metabolism and cellularity. *Clin Res, 15*:323, 1967.

Winick, M; Noble, A: Cellular response with increased feeding in neonatal rats. *J Nutr, 91*:176, 1967.

Adipose cell size and number in experimental human obesity. *Nutr Rev, 30*:60, 1972.

MODIFICATIONS IN CONSTITUENTS: A. PROTEIN*

I. INCREASED PROTEIN DIET

A HIGH PROTEIN DIET provides an additional amount of amino acids for replacement of body tissues depleted by increased losses or by inadequate protein intake. This diet includes approximately 125 grams of protein daily and provides about 1.6 grams protein per kilogram for a person weighing 70 kilograms.

Indications for Use

This diet is for people with protein depletion following a debilitating disease or condition; for those with neoplastic disease, extensive burns or blood loss, nephrotic syndrome, or cirrhosis of the liver without need for sodium restriction.

Diet Plan

The provision of 125 grams of protein may be accomplished by the addition of 2 cups of milk and 3 ounces of meat to the hospital General Diet making the total of these two foods for the day 4 cups of milk and 9 exchanges from the Meat Group. Since no maximum limits are set, and since additional protein will usually be obtained from other foods, the protein level will often be above 125 grams daily. Fat and carbohydrate are not limited.

The two diets with increased calories as listed is the preceding section are also high in protein and may be appropriate for those people who need exceptionally high levels of calories along with increased protein. No unusual foods or special ingredients are included in these diets.

---

*Margaret Newton, MD, Assoc Director Dialysis Unit, Univ of Wisconsin Center for Health Sciences, served as consultant.

101

Diet in Health and Disease

II. DECREASED PROTEIN DIETS

Protein Restriction Only

Protein foods of high biological value (from animal sources)

TABLE VI-1

DIET RESTRICTED IN PROTEIN ONLY

Protein 40 to 45 grams; No Electrolyte Restriction
Protein Values from Food Exchange System, Section II

Food Group	Amount	Protein (gm)
Milk	1 cup	8
Meat Group (including egg)	3 exchanges	21
Vegetable:		
List 2A, page 16	2 servings	0
List 2B, page 17	2 exchanges	4
Fruit, fruit juices	5 to 6 exchanges	0
Bread, cereals	3 exchanges	6
Non-protein foods: fats, honey, syrups, sugar, jelly, jam, etc.	As desired	0
	Total	39 gm

For a 45 gm protein diet, not restricted in electrolytes, add one of the following:
—1 egg
—1 cup ice cream
—3/4 exchange from the Milk Group

TABLE VI-2

CALCULATED NUTRIENT ESTIMATES OF DIETS WITH INCREASED OR RESTRICTED PROTEIN AS SERVED IN A HOSPITAL

Nutrients	Unit	Recommended Dietary Allowances Man 51+ Years Old	Woman 51+ Years Old	Hospital Increased Protein Diet	Hospital Increased Protein Diet
Food energy	Kcal	2,400	1,800	2,785	1,500
Protein	gm	56	46	128	40
Fat	gm	—	—	128	50
Carbohydrate	gm	—	—	286	235
Calcium	gm	0.8	0.8	1.8	0.6
Phosphorus	gm	0.8	0.8	2.2	0.7
Iron	mg	10	10	16.7	12
Magnesium	mg	350	300	385	222
Sodium	mg	—	—	4,481	1,446
Sodium mEq	mg			195	63
Potassium	mg	—	—	3,915	2,452
Potassium mEq	mg			100	63
Vitamin A	IU	5,000	4,000	7,666	8,929
Vitamin E activity		15 IU	12 IU	8.1 mg	6.5 mg
Ascorbic acid	mg	45	45	85	125
Folic acid	mg	0.4	0.4	—	—
Niacin equivalent	mg	16.0	12.0	39	16
Riboflavin	mg	1.5	1.1	3.2	1.1
Thiamin	mg	1.2	1.0	2.0	0.9
Vitamin B_6	mg	2.0	2.0	2.2	1.1
Vitamin B_{12}	mcg	3.0	3.0	8.5	1.6

are emphasized in the restricted protein diets. These foods contain the essential amino acids in the approximate amounts needed by the body. It is recommended that these foods be distributed throughout the meals of the day in order to provide for good utilization of the amino acids present and to prevent catabolism of body protein in excess of their anabolic rate (i.e., prevent a negative nitrogen balance).

III. CONTROLLED PROTEIN— CONTROLLED ELECTROLYTE DIETS FOR PATIENTS WITH RENAL DISEASE

Diets for patients with acute or chronic renal disease are designed to minimize protein catabolism and provide optimal nutrition in the face of a decreasing ability to regulate the renal excretion of end products of metabolism. They are intended to contain water, electrolytes, and vitamins sufficient to cover the amounts excreted by the diseased kidneys.

Urea, creatinine, uric acid, and ammonium salts are the main breakdown products of protein normally excreted in the urine. Their excretion is gradually reduced as renal function deteriorates, despite the fact that the diseased kidney has some ability to adapt by increasing the excretory rate per unit of functioning nephron. These substances are referred to as non-protein nitrogen (NPN) products.

Urea accounts for the largest proportion of NPN, the concentration increasing as kidney function deteriorates. When urea levels become abnormally high, gastrointestinal symptoms such as nausea, vomiting, and sometimes diarrhea develop. A low protein diet will lower the blood urea and thereby minimize or eliminate these symptoms in chronic uremia until the renal function gets below 5-10 percent of normal, at which time hemodialysis is required to assist in the removal of these substances. When a patient's condition is stabilized on regular dialysis, dietary protein content can be increased to normal or near normal, depending on the frequency and efficiency of dialysis. This can be accomplished without causing recurrence of nausea and vomiting.

Laboratory Tests

The most convenient and clinically useful measurements of

Diet in Health and Disease

renal function are the creatinine (Cr) and blood urea nitrogen (BUN), and their clearance rates. Clearances are defined as the amount of blood completely cleared of a blood constituent such as creatinine or urea as it passes through the kidney. The formula is:

$$C \text{ (Clearance of substance A)} = \frac{U \left\{\begin{matrix}\text{Concentration of}\\ \text{A in urine}\end{matrix}\right\} \times V \left\{\begin{matrix}\text{Volume of}\\ \text{urine per minute}\end{matrix}\right\}}{P \left\{\begin{matrix}\text{Concentration of}\\ \text{A in plasma}\end{matrix}\right\}}$$

or

$$C \text{ of substance A} = \frac{UV \text{ (in ml/min.)}}{P}$$

Normal creatinine clearance which indicates glomerular filtration rate (GFR) is approximately 120 to 140 ml/min for adult males and 100 to 120 ml/min for adult females, per 1.73 m^2 body surface. Since creatinine is secreted in small amounts by the renal tubules, the values are slightly higher than true GFR, but this test is used most commonly because it is easy to perform. True GFR can be measured by inulin clearance when necessary but it is much more costly and time consuming. Inulin is an exogenous substance which is neither reabsorbed nor secreted by the tubules. Patients *may* be asymptomatic until their GFR falls below 10 to 15 percent of normal.

Urea clearance values are slightly lower than true GFR because, although urea is freely filtered by the renal glomeruli, it is slightly reabsorbed by the renal tubules. In advanced uremia (5 to 15 percent of normal GFR) the true GFR can be obtained by averaging the urea and creatinine clearance, without performing the more complicated inulin clearance.

Blood concentrations of nitrogenous end products of metabolism rise as the clearance rates fall. For example, using creatinine clearances (C_{cr}) as a measure of GFR and plasma creatinine (Cr_{plasma}), the following ratios exist:

Creatinine Clearance	Plasma Creatinine
100 ml/min	1.0 mg/100 ml
50 ml/min	2.0 mg/100 ml
25 ml/min	4.0 mg/100 ml
12 ml/min	8.0 mg/100 ml
6 ml/min	16.0 mg/100 ml

Urea levels are influenced by the quantity of protein in the diet. Creatinine represents products that are influenced by cell turnover. The clinician translates these values into estimates of glomerular filtration rate as shown for creatinine.

Maximum blood urea clearance is given by Davidsohn and Henry (1969) as 64 to 99 ml per min, standard clearance (more than 75 percent of normal) as 41 to 65 ml per min. Normal blood urea nitrogen (BUN) ranges from 6 to 22 mg per 100 ml of plasma. Normal urea nitrogen of urine is 6 to 17 gm per 24 hours. To convert urea nitrogen to urea, multiply by 2.14 (Davidsohn and Henry, 1969).

Creatinine clearance from the blood is listed by the same authors as 117 ± 20 ml per minute or 150 to 180 liters per 24 hours. Normal creatinine level in serum is 0.5 to 1.2 mg per 100 ml (Davidsohn and Henry, 1969).

Electrolytes

The average daily intake of sodium chloride is given by the National Research Council (NAS-NRC, 1968) as 6 to 18 gm per day. This equals 2.4 to 7.5 gm sodium. Calculation of sodium intakes of persons securing a higher proportion of their calories from canned soups, cold meats, convenience foods and snack foods indicate that levels for some individuals may be considerably higher (Gormican, 1972).

Sodium concentration in the blood exerts an influence on the body's water balance. Sodium is the chief cation of extracellular fluid and plasma. Normal output of sodium in the urine ranges from 5 to 260 mEq/24 hours, varying with intake. Renal sodium excretion is not calculated as a "clearance" because almost all of the sodium filtered by the renal glomeruli is reabsorbed, the amount in the urine reflecting the dietary intake in healthy individuals taking no drugs which could alter the renal sodium excretion.

Interpretation of serum sodium concentration must take into account the state of hydration of the patient. For example, a patient who is severely dehydrated but with a normal serum sodium concentration is obviously sodium depleted and requires the administration of both salt and water in isosmotic quantities to restore his vascular and extracellular volumes to normal. Conversely an over-hydrated and edematous patient with a normal serum sodium has an excess of sodium and water in his extracellular, and possibly vascular, spaces. Sodium and water restriction, and possibly diuretics, are needed here despite normal concentration of serum sodium. Abnormally high or low serum sodiums must be evaluated accordingly.

As kidney function deteriorates, the kidney's range of sodium excretory capacity becomes less flexible. Hence the sodium intake will have to vary with this changing capacity to eliminate sodium. Some patients with renal disease have very high excretion rates of sodium and water which cannot, and should not, be reduced by dietary manipulation. Other renal patients, such as those with the nephrotic syndrome, may retain sodium avidly, and they require both sodium restricted diets and diuretics to promote greater sodium excretion.

The National Research Council (NAS-NRC, 1974) gives the average daily intake of potassium as between 50 and 150 mEq (1.95 to 5.85 gm). Davidsohn and Henry (1969) list normal plasma averages as 4.0 to 4.8 mEq per liter. Normal urine output of potassium is 40 to 80 mEq per 24 hours. The kidney maintains its ability to excrete potassium normally until the GFR is 10 to 15 percent, at which point the dietary intake must be restricted.

Other minerals, particularly calcium, phosphorus, magnesium, iron, copper, sulfur, and zinc are important in the medical management of renal disease, but they are practically never under quantitative dietary control. Phosphorus and vitamin D are being studied (Bricker, et al, 1969) so phosphorus exchanges are included in Table VI-5. Urinary phosphate excretion is impaired in advanced renal failure causing high serum phosphate values. Drugs which bind dietary phosphate preventing intestinal absorption, such as aluminum hydroxide, are generally used to control the rise in serum phosphate.

Water

Control of water intake becomes essential when the diseased kidneys can no longer regulate extracellular fluid volume, maintain acid-base balance and excrete toxic substances.

Zintel (in Wohl and Goodhart, 1968, Chap 34) summarizes water intake and output as follows:

Intake by mouth, daily:

Liquids	800 to 1500 ml
"Solid" food	1000 to 1500 ml
Oxidation of food- stuffs (Metabolic water)	200 to 400 ml
Total	2000 to 3400 ml

Output, daily:

Urine	850 to 1500 ml
Feces	150 ml
From skin and lungs (Insensible loss)	1000 to 1500 ml
Total	2000 to 3150 ml

Loss from vomiting, diarrhea, drainage, excessive sweating, etc., will be in addition to this. Daily weight loss or gain above an expected level is also a general indication of fluid balance. Rapid weight gain is associated with edema; rapid loss with dehydration.

Alper (in Wohl and Goodhart, 1968, Chap 12) gives the basis for an estimate of metabolic water (water from the oxidation of protein, fat, and carbohydrate) and notes that a range of values as follows is found in the literature:

	Metabolic water per gm
Protein	0.39 to 0.41 gm
Fat	1.07 gm
Carbohydrate	0.36 to 0.60 gm

When fluid restriction is required, the amount prescribed is in terms of milliliters or cubic centimeters per day. General hospital practice, when fluids are controlled, is to keep a bedside record of all liquids ingested. This includes water, ice, flavored drinks, juices, coffee, tea, milk, soup, ice cream, gelled desserts (all foods liquid at body temperature).

As urine output decreases and water control becomes more rigid, foods which are 80 to 95 percent water (mainly fruits and vegetables, and notably melons and tomatoes) are closely controlled. The water content of foods may require calculation. All foods contain some water. For instance, flour is about 12 percent water, breads 25 to 35 percent, cooked meats 50 to 75 percent and vegetables 75 to 95 percent. Watt and Merrill (1963) list the water content of foods. A rough estimate used in routine water calculation is the difference between the total weight of food and the sum of the weights of protein, fat, and carbohydrate. Fiber and minerals do not need to be considered in the water calculation. Patients with markedly reduced urine output generally require peritoneal dialysis or hemodialysis to remove excess water, electrolytes, and nitrogenous breakdown products.

Water and Chemical Sources of Electrolytes

If the diet prescription limits sodium and potassium severely, distilled water should be used for drinking and food preparation. Chemically-softened water should not be used. Tsaltas (1969) gave a method for leaching potassium from vegetables by using an excess of cooking water and gave a table of values on the leached product. Other nutrients are undoubtedly leached by this process, including water-soluble vitamins.

Water supplies vary in their electrolyte content and should be checked periodically. Information on the electrolyte content of the local water supply can be secured from the Water Supply Division (or similar name) of state department of natural resources. Generally, distilled water is used for sodium restricted diets if the local supply contains more than 1 mEq sodium per liter.

Descaling additives put into steam generating equipment can introduce chemicals into foods if direct steam connections are used. Present plumbing standards call for "clean steam" generating equipment at the site of use.

Direct steam has been used by some food processors. State standards define allowable water conditioning additives for this purpose. Chemicals have been injected into water used in ice machines to make clear ice and prevent mineral deposits in the lines and ice bins.

Dietary Modifications for Renal Patients

Dietary care of patients with renal disease depends upon the state of their disease and the availability of treatment by dialysis. The presence or absence of clinical signs and symptoms, their rate of development and severity, and the results of blood and urine analyses necessitate individualized treatment

In the early phase of chronic renal disease the patient can excrete water and metabolic products normally, so restrictions are seldom needed. Emphasis at this time is given to adequate nutrition and ideal body weight.

As the disease progresses, one or more physiologic abnormalities occur:

Impairment of excretion of breakdown products such as urea, resulting in abnormally high plasma values.

Impaired water excretion: it may increase in moderately advanced renal failure, and decrease during dehydration or terminal renal failure or temporary oliguric states.

Impaired sodium and potassium excretion. Obligatory sodium excretion may be very high during moderately advanced renal insufficiency with inability of the kidney to significantly increase or decrease its sodium and water losses. In oliguric or anuric phases of renal disease, sodium loss may be minimal or absent. The kidney can usually excrete normal dietary intake of potassium until the chronically diseased kidney has less than 10 to 15 percent of its normal GFR. Then excretion is reduced and dietary potassium must be lowered accordingly.

In acute renal disease, one or more of these symptoms come on rapidly. In chronic renal disease they develop more slowly.

In acute renal failure, oliguria (less than 400 ml urine per day) or anuria (less than 100 ml urine per day) may intervene. This life threatening situation requires strict dietary control of water, protein and electrolytes. Attempts are made to balance water and electrolyte intake and output. If the patient in this situation is being dialyzed, his diet can be substantially liberalized.

In oliguria and anuria protein restriction will slow the build-up of blood urea nitrogen. The degree of protein restriction required depends upon the percentage of renal dysfunction and whether or not the patient is being dialyzed. In anuria without dialysis all forms of protein are temporarily eliminated. Formerly, protein-free, essentially electrolyte-free sugar-fat mixtures were used to supply carbohydrate and calories during anuria. These were not well accepted by patients and poorly tolerated. Merrill (in Strauss and Welt, 1971) observes that their use is "now outmoded," largely because of the availability of hemodialysis. He suggests that small amounts of Karo syrup in gingerale, equal proportions, given frequently are as well tolerated as any supplement. Protein-free, electrolyte-free, high caloric supplements are available.

Mitchell and Smith (1966) recommended a protein intake of 0.2 to 0.5 gm protein per kg body weight for the patient on dialysis with oliguria. They limited fluid intake to the equivalent of insensible losses, and urine output, plus allowable weight gain between dialysis. Uremic patients dialyzed three times per week can safely ingest 80 grams of protein daily; this level is nutritionally advantageous.

Giordano (1963), and Giovannetti and Maggiore (1964) of Italy working independently developed the concept of using a minimum quantity of protein of high biological value (HBV) in the treatment of renal disease. Berlyne (1968) reviewed their work and adapted their diets to British tastes. Hegsted in the same publication described the biological value of different protein foods. He listed milk and eggs as superior to meat and legumes in providing essential amino acids in the ratios needed.

Seldin, Carter, and Rector (in Strauss and Welt, 1972, Chap 6) reviewed the historical development of low protein diets in renal disease. They note that a 40 gm protein diet is usually prescribed when the filtration rate falls below 20 ml per minute. They state that the protein content of the diet influences the magnitude of azotemia and the development of hyperkalemia and acidosis.

For the patient requiring a low electrolyte, low protein diet, Levin and Winklestein (1967) prepared an electrodialyzed whey formula which supplied 27 gm of protein and 377 calories per 100 gm. Karp (1971) developed formulas for other foods using the low electrolyte whey. Sorenson (1970) and Smith (1971) perfected gluten-free bread formulas for patients with uremia. See Appendix IV for lists of commercial companies selling gluten-free, low electrolyte products. Most of these companies also furnish recipes and other information. De St Joer (1970), Krawitt and Weinberger (1971), and Margie (1972) have compiled recipe books for patients on low protein diets.

Chronic Renal Failure With Dialysis

With prolongation of life through hemodialysis in chronic renal failure, emphasis has shifted from the minimum amino acids essential to maintain nitrogen balance to the use of a higher protein diet which will provide more minerals, vitamins, and calories in a form acceptable to the patient. Vitamin and calorie needs are increased.

Giordano, et al (1968) using the Travenal Kidney found that between 2.3 and 3.3 gm of amino acids were lost per hour, 14 to 20 gms including peptides, during a 6 hour dialysis. They stated that a low protein diet is contra-indicated in patients subject to frequent dialysis; it will hasten amino acids depletion and invite infection.

Comty (1968) reviewed the dietary requirements during dialysis and recommended a protein allowance of 1 gm per kg ideal body weight, plus an allowance to replace amino acid loss in the dialysate. She estimated a 20 gm protein loss.

Caloric intake is vital to conserve body protein. For a moderately active young adult Comty recommended 43 calories per kg for men and 41 calories per kg for women. She reported success with diets allowing up to 50 mEq sodium and 1000 ml measured fluid.

Kopple, et al (1969) on the basis of nitrogen balance studies on dialyzed patients found that at least 0.75 gm protein per kg was essential to replace nitrogen loss during dialysis; of this amount, 85 percent or 0.63 gm per kg was of high biologic value. Due to poor adherence to the diet at this level they recommended allowing 0.8 to 0.9 gm protein per kg of which 0.63 gm per kg was of high biologic value, and at least 35 calories per kg.

Maddox (in de St Joer, 1970) pointed out that if a patient is expected to purchase locally available foods, a diet of at least 60 gm protein per day will be required. Below this protein allowance special wheat starch flour and recipes would be required for adequate calories. This would materially increase the cost and decrease the convenience of the diet. He recommended vitamin supplementation and 45 calories per kg body weight.

Mackenzie (1971) reviewed the research on nutrition and nutritional losses during hemodialysis and made suggestions as to levels of nutrients in the dialysate.

Applegate (1972) outlined goals in the dietary treatment of the patient on intermittent dialysis:

1. As little restriction as possible within the limits of the dialysis program
2. Palatability
3. Variety
4. Individuality
5. Programmed splurges (as planned with the dietitian!)
6. Psychological manipulation giving the patient maximum freedom of choice

He gave specific criteria for evaluating the adequacy of dialysis:

1. Pre-dialysis BUN between 70 and 100 mg %
2. Pre-dialysis creatinine of 15 mg % or less
3. Potassium: pre-dialysis 6 mEq/L; post-dialysis 2.5 mEq/L
4. Phosphorus: pre-dialysis 7 mEq/L; post dialysis 2.5 mEq/L
5. Pre-dialysis blood pressure 150/100
6. Average hematocrit—not less than 18%
7. Inter-dialysis weight gain—4 lbs
8. Serum albumin—3.5 gm %
9. Serum iron—50 mcgm % (serum iron in the uremic patient is not a good indicator of whether the patient is iron deficient)
10. Improvement or stability of neuropathy
11. Return to ideal weight
12. No vomiting, headache or pruritis

Merrill recommends maintaining the hematocrit between 25 and 30 (in Strauss and Welt, 1971, page 659).

Low-Protein—Controlled Electrolyte Diet

Foods included in this diet are selected from Table VI-5.* The food groups in this table are similar to the food exchanges in Section I, but are grouped on the basis of protein and potassium content. Average sodium, phosphorus and calories of each group are given. Most diets will require control of protein and potassium only. Hence sodium, phosphorus and caloric values which are out of line with the others in the group are bracketed [ ]. Such foods would not be used if that nutrient were limited. Average values for sodium, phosphorus and calories do not include the bracketed items.

In setting up these tables, the lists originally formulated at Mount Sinai Hospital and revised by the Dietary Department of Cedars-Sinai Hospital of Los Angeles were used as models.

To some extent, frequency of use has been considered in grouping foods. Thus shellfish are not included with the meat exchange. The milk group is divided into three lists with List 3 (cream, cream cheese, and frozen desserts) in units of use, rather than quantities adjusted to the level of one cup of milk.

The protein values of meat, poultry, and fish in these lists are

---

*Weights of household measures of these foods as shown in the tables are from Home and Garden Bulletin 72: *Nutritive Value of Food* (1970), *Average Weight of a Measured Cup of Various Foods* by Dawson, Gilpin, and Fulton (ARS 61-6, 1969), and *Handbook of Food Preparation* (Amer Home Econ Assoc, 1971).

the same as the protein value of the Lean Meat List. Vegetables in List 1 and List 2, Table VI-5, are selected to provide potassium at the levels of 4 and 6 mEq respectively. The portion (weight) is adjusted to provide the amount of potassium designated as the average for each list. Fruits are divided into six lists ranging up to 0.5 mEq potassium above or below the given value of the range. The average of each group, not adjusted for frequency of use, very closely approximates the rounded value assigned to the group. Except for List 1, Table VI-5, all fruits are in 100 gm portions. However, that does not equal 1/2 cupful for all items.

"Regular" is used in these tables to describe foods that are prepared either at home or commercially without any modification for dietetic purpose. Foods that are prepared without added salt may also be designated as "salt-free" or "SF." Foods canned without salt are so noted; otherwise they are the standard commercial pack. Labels should be checked because of the rapidly changing condition of the market. Particular attention should be given to ingredients containing potassium or sodium. "Diet" or "dietetic" foods may have sodium and potassium in the additives. Laws regarding allowable ingredients in commercially processed foods vary from state to state. When potassium is limited in the diet all low sodium preparations should be checked for potassium content before being used. The sodium and potassium content of some salt substitutes and of low sodium baking powders are included in Table VI-7.

"Special" refers to foods especially prepared to meet the needs of one or more dietary restriction. In this section the term refers to foods prepared from ingredients selected for their low protein, low electrolyte content. Certain items made with wheat starch or a low protein, low electrolyte baking mix are referred to by specific names such as "wheat starch bread" or "gluten-free bread." Low protein pastas are available (see Appendix IV).

Dehydrated and "instant" foods are not included in the low-protein, low-potassium tables. They vary widely in the kind and amount of additives; also processors' formulas change.

If sodium is restricted, foods should be cooked and served without added salt. Salt substitutes which are chiefly potassium salts should not be used. The potassium content of selected medicines, foods, and salt substitutes is given by RE Pearson and KH Fish, Jr, in *Hospital Pharmacy, 6* (no 9):6, 1971.

TABLE VI-3

BASIC PLAN OF DIET: PROTEIN 40 gm, POTASSIUM 40 mEq

Values and Portions of Foods from Table VI-5.
No salt added.

	Measure	Weight	Protein gm	Potassium mEq	Sodium mEq	Phosphorus mEq	Calories
Milk Group							
Milk, whole	½ cup	122	4.1	4.5	2.7	6.6	80
Half and half	¼ cup	60	1.9	2.0	1.2	3.0	80
Meat Exchanges	3 exchanges	See list	24.0	8.1	3.0	12.3	165
Eggs, 3 in a week	3/7 egg		2.6	0.7	1.1	2.6	34
Breads-Cereals							
Wheat starch bread	¼ loaf	See list	0.5	0.4	1.6	—	435
Cereal: SF grain food, List 2	1 exchange	See list	2.0	0.7	0	0.2	70
Subtotals			35.1	16.4	9.6	26.5	846
Vegetables							
List 1	1 exchange	See list	1.0	4.0	0.3	1.5	20
List 2	1 exchange	See list	2.0	6.0	0.3	2.1	25
Fruits							
List 2	1 exchange	See list	0.5	2.0	0	0.5	65
List 3	1 exchange	See list	0.5	3.0	0	0.8	70
List 6	1 exchange	See list	0.5	6.0	0.2	0.8	60
List 1	1 exchange	See list	0	1.0	0	0.3	Variable
Totals			39.6	38.4	10.5	32.5	1086

Fats, Oils, and Sweets   See lists. As desired to add calories and palatability. Other combinations of fruits and vegetables to provide approximately 5 gm protein and 23 mEq potassium can be used. Common practice allows slight deviations. If sodium is not restricted, salt can be added in cooking and serving.

Coffee, tea, or decaffeinated beverages are not indicated in the meal plans in this section but may be used subject to the physician's direction. They should be recognized as a source of considerable potassium and the diet prescription modified sufficiently to allow a controlled amount. They are not calculated in the basic plan for these reasons:

1. Electrolytes in the prepared beverage depend on the water supply, the equipment used, and the length of time of preparation.
2. Values for electrolytes in instant coffee and tea in Handbook no 8

TABLE VI-4

SUMMARY: PROTEIN-POTASSIUM-SODIUM EXCHANGES
IN PROTEIN-POTASSIUM-CONTROLLED DIETS

Assigned values of exchange lists. Protein, Potassium and Calorie values are rounded averages.

	Portion	Protein gm	Potassium mEq	Sodium mEq	Phosphorus mEq	Calories
Milk, fluid	1 exchange	8.5	9.0	5.3	13.2	160
Cheese	1 exchange	8.0	0.8	— — — Variable — — —		
Meat, poultry, fish, cooked	1 exchange	8.0	2.7	1.0	4.1	55
Egg	One, 8/lb	6.0	1.7	2.7	6.0	80
Vegetables:						
List 1	1 exchange	1.0	4.0	0.3	1.5	20
List 2	1 exchange	2.0	6.0	0.3	2.1	25
Fruits:						
List 1	1 exchange	(0)	1.0	(0)	0.3	Variable
List 2	1 exchange	0.5	2.0	(0)	0.5	65
List 3	1 exchange	0.5	3.0	0.1	0.8	70
List 4	1 exchange	0.5	4.0	0.1	0.8	55
List 5	1 exchange	1.0	5.0	0.2	0.8	60
List 6	1 exchange	0.5	6.0	0.2	0.8	45
Grain Foods:						
List 1, Low protein, and special products	Not an exchange list. Individual values are given.					
List 2, Low protein, low potassium, low sodium	1 exchange	2.0	0.7	(0)	2.0	70
List 3, Moderate sodium, regular	See list in Table VI-5					
Fats, Oils:						
Salt-free butter, margarine	1 tbsp	(0)	(0)	(0)	0.1	100
Salt-free mayonnaise	1 tbsp	(0)	0.1	(0)	0.2	100
Oils, shortenings	1 tbsp	0	0	0	0	115
Sweets, List 1	1 tbsp	0	0.2	0.2	0.1	50
Miscellaneous	See lists					

TABLES VI-5—FOODS USED IN PROTEIN AND ELECTROLYTE RESTRICTED DIETS
PROTEIN-POTASSIUM-SODIUM EXCHANGE LISTS, AND PROTEIN AND ELECTROLYTES IN SELECTED FOODS

Protein value used in exchanges rounded to multiples of 0.5 gm. Calorie value used in exchanges rounded to nearest multiple of 5. Values in brackets not included in averages. Salt added in cooking or serving not included in values.

MILK GROUP

List 1 Fluid Milk Exchanges[1]

Value: Protein 8.5 gm   Sodium 122 mg (5.3 mEq)   Calories variable
Potassium 351 mg (9 mEq)   Phosphorus 229 mg (13.2 mEq)

	Portion Measure	Weight gm	Protein gm	Potassium mg	Potassium mEq	Sodium mg	Sodium mEq	Phosphorus mg	Phosphorus mEq	Calories
Buttermilk	1 cup	245	8.8	343	8.8	[319]	[13.8]	233	13.5	88
Chocolate milk drink made with skim milk	1 cup	250	8.3	355	9.1	115	5.0	228	13.3	197
Milk, whole, 3.5% fat	1 cup	244	8.5	351	9.0	122	5.3	227	13.2	160
Milk, skim	1 cup	245	8.8	355	9.1	127	5.5	233	13.5	90
Milk partially skimmed, fortified with 2% solids	4/5 cup	200	8.4	350	9.0	122	5.3	224	13.0	118
Yogurt from partially skimmed milk	1 cup	245	8.5	350	9.0	125	5.4	230	13.4	125
Averages for List I, Fluid Milk			8.5	351	9.0	122	5.3	229	13.3	130

List 2 Cheese Exchanges

Value: Protein 8 gm   Sodium variable   Calories variable
Potassium 32 mg (0.8 mEq)   Phosphorus variable

	Weight gm	Protein gm	Potassium mg	Potassium mEq	Sodium mg	Sodium mEq	Phosphorus mg	Phosphorus mEq	Calories
Cheese, cheddar, natural	28	7.0	23	0.6	[196]	[8.5]	136	7.8	115
Cottage cheese, creamed	¼ cup	61	8.3	52	1.3	140	6.1	74	4.3	130
Cottage cheese, uncreamed	¼ cup	50	9.0	36	0.9	145	6.3	88	5.1	40
Processed American cheese	28	7.0	22	0.6	[318]	[13.8]	[432]	[25.1]	105
Swiss cheese, domestic	28	8.0	28	0.7	[327]	[14.2]	[315]	[18.3]	105
Averages for List 2, Cheeses		7.9	32	0.8	variable		variable		variable

List 3   Cream, Cream Cheese and Frozen Desserts² | Not exchanges |

		Weight gm	Protein gm	Potassium mg	mEq	Sodium mg	mEq	Phosphorus mg	mEq	Calories
Cream:										
20% fat	2 Tbsp	30	0.9	37	1.0	13	0.6	24	1.4	63
Light whipping, 31% fat	2 Tbsp	30	0.8	31	0.8	11	0.5	20	1.2	90
Heavy whipping, 38% fat	2 Tbsp	30	0.7	27	0.7	10	0.4	18	1.0	99
Cream cheese	1 oz	28	2.3	21	0.5	71	3.1	27	1.6	106
Half and half, 12% fat	¼ cup	60	1.9	77	2.0	28	1.2	51	3.0	80
Ice cream:										
10% fat	½ cup	62	2.8	122	3.1	39	1.7	71	4.1	119
12% fat	½ cup	62	2.5	69	1.8	25	1.1	61	3.5	128
Ice Milk, soft serve	½ cup	88	4.2	171	4.4	60	2.6	109	6.3	134
Sherbet, orange	½ cup	82	0.8	18	0.5	8	0.3	11	0.6	108

¹If additional calories are needed, add fat when low fat milks are used.

²With adjustments in quantity to equivalent protein value, frozen desserts can be used in exchanges for milk to increase the calorie value of the diet. Cream can be exchanged on an equivalent weight basis for milk without diet adjustment for protein and electrolytes.

MEAT, POULTRY, FISH, EGGS
(For Legumes and Nuts See Table VI-7)

List 1   Meat Exchanges | Value: Protein 8.0 gm   Phosphorus 71 mg (4.1 mEq)   Calories 55
Potassium 103 mg (2.7 mEq)   Sodium 22 mg (1.0 mEq)

	Weight of One Exchange		Protein	Potassium		Sodium		Phosphorus		Calories
	oz	gm	gm	mg	mEq	mg	mEq	mg	mEq	
Meats, lean only, cooked										
Hamburger, cooked	1	28	7.8	104	2.7	17	0.7	65	3.8	61
Pot roast	1	28	8.4	104	2.7	17	0.7	42	2.4	62
Round, broiled	1	28	8.9	104	2.7	17	0.7	76	4.4	54
Sirloin, broiled	1	28	9.0	104	2.7	17	0.7	71	4.1	48
Ham, lightly cured	1	28	7.2	92	2.4	[260]	[11.3]	57	3.3	52
Lamb: leg, loin	1	28	8.0	82	2.1	20	0.9	67	3.9	52

MEAT, POULTRY, FISH, EGGS (Continued)

	Weight of One Exchange		Protein	Potassium		Sodium		Phosphorus		Calories
	oz	gm	gm	mg	mEq	mg	mEq	mg	mEq	
Liver, beef, fried	1	28	7.4	107	2.7	52	2.2	135	7.8	64
Pork, fresh: leg, loin, shoulder, spareribs	1	28	8.0	109	2.8	18	0.8	83	4.8	67
Veal, round, broiled	1	28	7.7	140	3.6	22	1.0	65	3.8	60
Average			8.0	105	2.7	2	1.0	73	4.3	58
Poultry, roasted, no skin										
Chicken	1	28	8.7	105	2.7	21	0.9	62	3.6	48
Turkey	1	28	8.8	104	2.7	36	1.6	65	3.8	53
Average			8.8	104	2.7	28	1.3	64	3.7	51
Fish										
Cod, flounder, haddock, halibut, cooked	1	28	6.2	112	2.9	40	1.7	73	4.2	45
Salmon, pink, canned without salt, solids and liquids	1	28	5.7	100	2.6	18	0.8	81	4.7	40
Tuna, canned water pack, salt free, solids and liquids	1	28	7.8	78	2.0	11	0.5	54	3.1	36
Average			6.5	97	2.5	23	1.0	69	4.0	40
Average Values for Meat, Poultry, Fish, List 1			7.8	103	2.7	22	1.0	71	4.1	53
List 2 Shellfish Not included in Meat Exchanges. If used frequently in place of above meat exchanges, diet will need adjustment.										
Clams, canned, solids and liquids	2½	70	5.5	98	2.5	—		96	5.1	37
Crab, canned	1½	42	7.3	46	1.2	[430]	[18.3]	76	4.4	42
Lobster, northern, canned or cooked	1½	42	7.9	76	1.9	[88]	[3.8]	81	4.7	27
Oysters, eastern, raw	3	85	7.1	103	2.6	62	2.7	121	7.1	57
Shrimp, raw	1½	42	7.6	92	2.4	59	2.6	70	4.1	38
List 3 Eggs										
Egg, 8 to lb	One egg	50	6.0	65	1.7	61	2.7	103	6.0	80
Egg, 3 per week	3/7 egg	21	2.6	28	0.7	26	1.1	44	2.6	34

VEGETABLE EXCHANGES

List 1 4 mEq POTASSIUM	Exchange Value: Protein 1.0 gm		Sodium 8 mg (0.3 mEq)						
	Potassium 156 mg (4 mEq)		Phosphorus 26 mg 1.5 mEq		Calories 20				
		Weight of	Weight to yield	Portion Adjusted to Provide 4 mEq Potassium					
Fresh and frozen items boiled and drained unless noted as raw	Potassium per 100 gms	one cup	156 mg Potassium	Measure	Protein	Sodium		Phosphorus		Calories
	mg	gm	gm	cup	gm	mg	mEq	mg	mEq	
Beans, lima, canned, SF	222	186	70	1/3	3.1	3	0.1	47	2.7	49
Beans, snap:										
Canned, SF	95	141	164	1	2.5	4	0.2	41	2.4	36
Fresh or frozen	152	161	103	2/3	1.5	1	(0)	31	1.8	28
Beets:										
Canned, sliced, SF	167	176	93	1/2	0.8	[43]	[1.9]	15	0.9	29
Fresh	208	205	75	1/3	0.8	[32]	[1.4]	17	1.0	24
Beet greens, fresh	332	145	47	1/3	0.8	[36]	[1.6]	12	0.7	8
Cabbage:										
Raw, shredded	233	63	67	1	0.9	13	0.6	19	1.1	16
Boiled	163	146	96	2/3	1.0	12	0.5	19	1.1	19
Cabbage, chinese, raw	253	59	61	1	0.7	14	0.6	40	2.3	9
Carrots:										
Raw, shredded	341	109	46	3/8	0.5	22	1.0	17	1.0	19
Fresh	222	153	70	1/2	0.6	23	1.0	22	1.3	22
Cauliflower:										
Raw	295	83	53	2/3	1.2	5	0.2	22	1.3	12
Fresh	206	179	76	1/2	1.7	7	0.3	36	2.1	17
Frozen	207	179	75	1/2	1.4	8	0.3	29	1.7	14
Chicory, green, raw, cut	420	53	37	2/3	0.4	—		15	0.9	7
Corn:										
WK, canned, solids & liquid, SF	97	256	161	5/8	3.1	3	0.1	[77]	[4.5]	[92]
Frozen	184	182	85	1/2	2.6	1	(0)	[62]	[3.6]	[67]

VEGETABLE EXCHANGES (Continued)

Fresh and frozen items boiled and drained unless noted as raw	Potassium per 100 gms mg	Weight of one cup gm	Weight to yield 156 mg Potassium gm	Portion Adjusted to Provide 4 mEq Potassium						
				Measure cup	Protein gm	Sodium mg	Sodium mEq	Phosphorus mg	Phosphorus mEq	Calories
Cucumbers, sliced, raw	160	144	98	2/3	0.6	6	0.3	18	1.0	14
Eggplant	150	201	104	1/2	1.0	1	(0)	22	1.3	20
Endive, curly, raw	294	48	53	1	0.9	7	0.3	29	1.7	11
Escarole, chopped, raw	294	48	53	1	0.9	7	0.3	29	1.7	11
Lettuce, raw:										
Butterhead	264	60	59	1 (9 leaves)	0.7	5	0.2	15	0.9	8
Crisphead	175	59	89	1-1/3	0.8	8	0.3	20	1.2	13
Looseleaf	264	60	59	1	0.5	5	0.2	13	0.8	11
Romaine	264	48	59	1	0.5	5	0.2	13	0.8	11
Mushrooms, raw, sliced	414	68	38	1/2	1.0	8	0.3	44	2.5	11
Mustard greens:										
Fresh	220	221	71	1/3	1.6	13	0.6	23	1.3	16
Frozen	157	114	100	1/2	1.2	10	0.4	43	2.5	20
Okra, fresh	174	160	89	1/2	3.0	3	0.1	[66]	[3.8]	46
Onions:										
Green, raw	231	99	68	2/3	1.1	5	0.2	39	2.3	45
Mature, raw, chopped	157	173	100	1/2	1.5	10	0.4	36	2.1	38
Mature, cut, boiled	110	179	142	3/4	1.7	10	0.4	41	2.4	41
Parsley, raw	727	64	21	1/3	0.8	9	0.4	13	0.8	9
Peas:										
Early June, cnd, drained sol, SF	96	172	163	1	[7.2]	5	0.2	[95]	[5.5]	[78]
Fresh	196	163	80	1/2	[4.3]	1	—	[79]	[4.6]	57
Frozen	135	167	115	2/3	[5.9]	[117]	[5.1]	[99]	[5.8]	[126]
Radishes, raw, whole	322	132	48	1/3	0.5	9	0.4	14	0.8	9

Food	Potassium (mg)			Measure	Protein (gm)	Sodium (mg)	Phosphorus (mg)	Calories		
Squash, summer, incl zucchini, fresh	141	238	110	1/2	1.0	1	—	27	1.6	15
Sweet potatoes, cnd, SF, no sugar	120	200	130	2/3	0.9	16	0.7	38	2.2	[60]
Turnip greens	149	163	107	2/3	2.7	18	0.8	41	2.4	25
Average Value					1.2	7	0.3	26	1.5	21

List 2 6 mEq POTASSIUM

	Exchange Value:	Protein 2.0 gm		Calories 25
	Potassium 234 mg (6 mEq)	Sodium 7 mg (0.3 mEq)	Phosphorus 36 mg (2.1 mEq)	

Food	Potassium (mg)	Measure	Protein (gm)	Sodium (mg)	Phosphorus (mg)	Calories		
Asparagus:								
Fresh	183	1/2 scant	1.7	1	(0)	39	2.3	16
Frozen, cuts	220	1/2	3.4	1	(0)	67	3.9	23
Frozen, spears	238	1/2	3.1	1	(0)	66	3.8	30
Broccoli:								
Fresh	267	1/2	2.7	9	0.4	55	3.2	23
Frozen spears	220	1/2	3.4	13	0.6	68	4.0	29
Brussels sprouts:								
Fresh	273	1/2	3.6	9	0.4	62	3.6	31
Frozen	295	1/2 scant	2.5	11	0.5	48	2.8	26
Celery:								
Fresh, raw, diced	341	2/3	0.6	[87]	[3.8]	19	1.1	12
Cooked	239	1/2	0.8	[86]	[3.7]	22	1.3	14
Chard, swiss	321	1/3	1.3	[63]	[2.7]	18	1.0	13
Collards:								
Fresh, leaves & stems	234	2/3	2.7	25	1.1	39	2.3	29
Frozen	236	2/3	2.9	16	0.7	51	3.0	30
Dandelion greens, fresh	232	2/3	2.0	[44]	[1.9]	42	2.4	33
Kale, leaves & stems	221	1/2	3.4	[47]	[2.0]	49	2.8	30
Peppers, sweet green, raw	213	2/3	1.3	14	0.6	24	1.4	24
Potatoes, white, pared	285	1 small	1.6	2	0.1	34	2.0	53

(See Table VI-7 for potatoes cooked in skin)

VEGETABLE EXCHANGES (Continued)

Fresh and frozen items boiled and drained unless noted as raw	Potassium per 100 gms	Weight of one cup	Weight to yield 234 mg Potassium	Portion Adjusted to Provide 6 mEq Potassium						
				Measure	Protein	Sodium		Phosphorus		Calories
	mg	gm	gm	cup	gm	mg	mEq	mg	mEq	
Pumpkin, canned	240	243	98	2/3	1.0	2	0.1	25	1.5	33
Rutabaga, fresh	167	163	140	3/4	1.3	6	0.3	43	2.5	49
Spinach:										
Fresh	324	156	72	1/2	2.2	[36]	[1.6]	27	1.6	17
Frozen leaf	362	156	64	1/2	1.9	[31]	[1.3]	28	1.6	15
Squash, winter, all varieties:										
Fresh	258	244	91	3/8	1.0	1	(0)	29	1.7	35
Frozen	207	241	113	1/2	1.4	1	(0)	36	2.1	43
Tomatoes:										
Fresh, raw	244	181	96	1/2	1.1	3	0.1	26	1.5	21
Canned, regular pack	217	238	108	1/2	1.1	[140]	[6.1]	26	1.5	23
Canned, SF	217	238	108	1/2	1.1	3	0.1	21	1.2	22
Tomato juice:										
Canned, regular pack	227	240	103	1/2	0.9	[206]	[9.0]	19	1.1	20
Canned, SF	227	240	103	1/2	0.8	3	0.1	19	1.1	20
Turnips, fresh	188	155	123	3/4	1.0	3	0.1	30	1.7	28
Average Value					1.9	7	0.3	36	2.1	26

FRUIT EXCHANGES

List 1　1 mEq POTASSIUM (Range 20-57 mg)

Exchange Value:　Protein (0)　　　　Sodium (0)　　　Calories Variable
Potassium 39 mg (1 mEq)　　Phosphorus 5 mg (0.3 mEq)

	Weight of Portion	Weight of one cup	Measure of Portion	Protein	Potassium	Sodium	Phosphorus	Calories
	gm	gm	cup	gm	mg	mg	mg	
Cranberry juice cocktail	200	250	4/5	0.2	20	2	6	130
Lemon juice	30	244	2 tbsp	(0)	42	(0)	3	1
Lemonade, conc froz, diluted x 4-1/3	248	248	1	0.4	40	(0)	3	111
Limeade, conc froz, diluted x 4-1/3	247	247	1	trace	32	(0)	3	103

Food	gm	(mg)	Measure	Protein	Potassium	(mEq)	Phosphorus	Calories
Blueberries, canned, heavy syrup	100	250	3/8	0.4	55	1	8	101
Grape juice, conc froz, diluted 1 to 3	100	253	3/8	0.2	34	1	4	53
Cranberries, fresh	60	114	1/2	0.2	49	1	6	28
Cranberry sauce, canned, strained	100	277	3/8	0.1	30	1	4	146
Cranberry orange relish	57	255	1/4	0.2	42	2	5	103
Pear nectar	125	250	1/2	0.4	49	1	6	65
Average Value				0.2	39	1	5	84

List 2   2 mEq POTASSIUM
(Range 58-97 mg)

Exchange Value: Protein 0.5 gm   Sodium (0)   Calories 65
Potassium 78 mg (2 mEq)   Phosphorus 9 mg (0.5 mEq)

Food	gm	(mg)	Measure	Protein	Potassium	(mEq)	Phosphorus	Calories
Applesauce, canned, sweetened	100	259	3/8	0.2	65	2	5	91
Blueberries:								
Raw, fresh	100	146	2/3	0.7	81	1	13	62
Frozen, sweetened	100	228	1/2	0.6	66	1	11	105
Frozen, unsweetened	100	165	2/3	0.7	81	1	13	55
Peach nectar	100	250	3/8	0.2	78	1	11	48
Pears, canned, light syrup	100	164	2/3	0.2	85	1	7	61
Pineapple, all styles, canned, light syrup	100	262	2/3	0.3	97	1	8	59
Pineapple-grapefruit drink	100	249	3/8	0.2	70	(0)	6	54
Average Value				0.4	78	1	9	67

List 3   3 mEq POTASSIUM
(Range 98-135 mg)

Exchange Value: Protein 0.5 gm   Sodium 2 mg (0.1 mEq)   Calories 70
Potassium 117 mg (3 mEq)   Phosphorus 14 mg (0.8 mEq)

Food	gm	(mg)	Measure	Protein	Potassium	(mEq)	Phosphorus	Calories
Apple, fresh, stored	100	248	1 small	0.2	110	1	10	60
Apple juice	100		3/8	0.1	101	1	9	47
Blackberries:								
Frozen, sweetened	100	252	2/3	0.6	66	1	11	105
Frozen, unsweetened	100	144	1/2	0.7	81	1	13	55
Cherries, red sour, pitted:								
Canned, water pack	100	215	3/8	0.8	130	2	13	43
Frozen, sweetened	100	259	1/2	1.0	130	2	15	112
Cherries, sweet, canned, heavy syrup	100	191	1/2	1.3	126	1	19	81

FRUIT EXCHANGES (Continued)

	Weight of Portion gm	Weight of one cup gm	Measure of Portion cup	Protein gm	Potassium mg	Sodium mg	Phosphorus mg	Calories
Grapefruit:								
Raw	100	226	3/8	0.5	135	1	16	41
Canned, syrup	100	256	3/8	0.6	135	1	14	70
Grape juice, canned or bottled	100	253	3/8	0.2	116	2	12	66
Orange apricot drink	100	249	3/8	0.5	94	(0)	8	50
Loganberries, canned, light syrup	100	240	3/8	0.7	111	1	11	70
Peaches								
Canned	100	255	3/8	0.4	133	2	13	58
Frozen, sweetened	100	236	3/8	0.4	124	2	13	88
Pears, raw	100	164	2/8	0.7	130	2	11	61
Pineapple, frozen, sweetened	100	246	3/8	0.4	100	2	4	85
Raspberries, frozen, sweetened	100	249	3/8	0.7	100	1	17	98
Strawberries, frozen, sliced, sweetened	100	254	3/8	0.5	112	1	17	109
Tangarines, fresh	100	193	1/2	0.8	126	2	18	46
Watermelon, fresh	100	160	2/3	0.5	111	6	19	26
Average Value				0.6	113	2	13	69

Exchange Value: Protein 0.5 gm; Sodium 2 mg (0.1 mEq); Potassium 156 mg (4 mEq); Phosphorus 14 mg (0.8 mEq); Calories 55

List 4   4 mEq POTASSIUM (Range 136-174 mg)

	Weight of Portion gm	Weight of one cup gm	Measure of Portion cup	Protein gm	Potassium mg	Sodium mg	Phosphorus mg	Calories
Apricot nectar	100	251	3/8	0.3	151	(0)	12	57
Blackberries:								
Raw	100	146	2/3	1.2	170	1	19	58
Frozen, unsweetened	100	252	3/8	1.2	153	1	24	48
Figs, canned, light syrup	100	253	3/8	0.5	152	2	13	65
Fruit cocktail:								
Canned, light syrup	100	256	3/8	0.4	164	5	12	60
Canned, water pack	100	256	3/8	0.4	168	5	13	37

Food	gm		Measure	Protein	Potassium	Sodium	Phosphorus	Calories
Grapefruit juice:								
Canned, unsweetened	100	247	3/8	0.5	162	1	14	41
Frozen, conc, sweetened, diluted 1 to 3	100	247	3/8	0.4	144	1	14	47
Grapes:								
American type, slip skin	100	153	2/3	1.3	158	3	12	69
European type, tight skin	100	160	2/3	0.6	173	3	20	67
Pineapple, raw	100	155	2/3	0.4	146	1	8	52
Pineapple-grapefruit drink	100	(245)	3/8	0.2	136	1	8	54
Pineapple juice:								
Canned, unsweetened	100	249	3/8	0.4	149	1	9	55
Frozen, conc, diluted 3 to 1	100	249	3/8	0.4	136	1	8	52
Plums, raw, sliced:								
Japanese and hybrid (all except Damson)	100	169	2/3	0.5	170	1	18	48
Prune type, halves	100	159	2/3	0.8	170	1	18	75
Plums, purple:								
Canned, water pack	100	245	3/8	0.4	148	2	10	46
Canned, light syrup	100	234	3/8	0.4	145	1	10	63
Raspberries, raw	100	144	2/3	1.2	168	1	22	57
Strawberries, raw	100	144	2/3	0.7	164	1	21	37
Average Value				0.6	152	2	14	55

List 5 5 mEq POTASSIUM (Range 175–214 mg)

Exchange Value: Protein 1.0 gm   Potassium 195 mg (5 mEq)   Sodium 5 mg (0.2 mEq)   Phosphorus 14 mg (0.8 mEq)   Calories 60

Food	gm		Measure	Protein	Potassium	Sodium	Phosphorus	Calories
Blackberries, raw	100	146	2/3	1.2	170	1	19	58
Cherries, sweet, raw	100	158	2/3	1.3	191	2	19	70
Grape juice, frozen	100	250	3/8	0.6	177	1	13	44
Grapefruit-orange juice, froz, diluted 1 to 3	100	(244)	3/8	0.6	177	1	13	44
Melon (cantaloup, honeydew):								
Frozen in syrup	100	231	1/2	0.6	188	9	12	62
Orange, raw, small	100	241	3/8	1.0	200	1	20	49

FRUIT EXCHANGES (Continued)

	Weight of Portion gm	Weight of one cup gm	Measure of Portion cup	Protein gm	Potassium mg	Sodium mg	Phosphorus mg	Calories
Orange juice:								
Fresh	100	244	3/8	0.7	200	1	17	45
Frozen conc, diluted 1 to 3	100	245	3/8	0.7	186	1	16	45
Peaches, raw, sliced	100	177	2/3	0.6	202	1	19	38
Rhubarb, cooked, sweetened	100	248	3/8	0.5	203	2	15	141
Average Value				0.8	189	2	16	60

List 6   6 mEq POTASSIUM
(Range 215-254 mg)

Exchange Value: Protein 0.5 gm   Sodium 5 mg (0.2 mEq)
Potassium 234 mg (6 mEq)   Phosphorus 14 mg (0.8 mEq)   Calories 45

	Weight of Portion gm	Weight of one cup gm	Measure of Portion cup	Protein gm	Potassium mg	Sodium mg	Phosphorus mg	Calories
Apricots, canned, light syrup	100	252	3/8	0.7	239	1	15	66
Muskmelons:								
Fresh cantaloup, casaba, honeydew	100	162	2/3	0.9	251	12	12	30
Papayas, fresh	100	182	1/2	0.6	234	3	16	39
Average Value				0.7	241	5	14	45

GRAIN FOODS

Not an exchange list

List 1   Low Protein and Special Products

	Portion Measure	Weight gm	Protein gm	Potassium mg	Potassium mEq	Sodium mg	Sodium mEq	Phosphorus mg	Phosphorus mEq	Calories
Cellu Low Protein Baking Mix		100	0.2	8	0.2	38	1.6	48	2.2	400
Cornstarch	1 tbsp	14	(0)	trace		(0)		(0)		51
Gluten-free cornstarch bread (Smith, 1971)	1 slice	25	0.5	21	0.5	1		—		68
Tapioca	1 tbsp	14	0.1	3	0.1	1		3		49

	Amount	gm	Protein gm	Potassium mg	Potassium mEq	Sodium mg	Sodium mEq	Phosphorus mg	Phosphorus mEq	Calories
Wheat starch, Paygel-P		100	0.3	7	0.2			6	0.3	350
Wheat starch bread, home baked (Sorenson, 1970)										
	1 loaf (20 slices)	525	1.9	58	1.5	148	6.4	(0)		1730
	1 slice	26	0.1	3	0.1	7	0.3	(0)		87

For all other low protein products made with wheat starch (such as pastas, muffins, crackers and desserts), see publications of suppliers of special dietary products, Appendix IV.

List 2 Low Potassium, Low Sodium Breads and Cereals

Exchange Value: Protein 2 gm   Potassium 26 mg (0.7 mEq)   Sodium 1 mg (0 mEq)   Phosphorus 39 mg (2.0 mEq)   Calories 70

Food	Amount	gm	Protein gm	Potassium mg	Potassium mEq	Sodium mg	Sodium mEq	Phosphorus mg	Phosphorus mEq	Calories
Bread, white, SF, local bakery (calculated values)	1 slice	25	2.0	15	0.4	4	0.2	18	1.1	66
Cornmeal, degermed	2 tbsp	20	1.6	24	0.6	(0)	(0)	20	1.2	72
Cream of rice, dry	2 tbsp	20	1.2	(0)	(0)	(0)	(0)	19	1.1	76
Farina, instant, dry	2 tbsp	20	2.3	17	0.4	1	(0)	79	4.6	72
Noodles, cooked	1/2 cup	80	3.3	35	0.9	2	0.1	42	2.4	96
Puffed rice, added nutrients, without salt	1 cup	15	0.9	15	0.4	(0)	(0)	18	1.1	60
Puffed wheat, added nutrients, without salt	1 cup	15	2.2	51	1.3	1	0.1	48	2.8	54
Rice, brown, dry	2 tbsp	20	1.5	43	1.1	2	0.1	44	2.5	72
Rice, white, dry	2 tbsp	20	1.3	18	0.5	1	(0)	19	1.1	73
Spaghetti, cooked till tender	1/2 cup	70	2.4	43	1.1	1	(0)	35	2.0	78
Averages for List 2		26	1.9	26	0.7	1	(0)	34	2.0	72

List 3 Low Potassium, Moderate Sodium Breads and Cereals, Regular

Can be used as protein-potassium exchanges for List 2 items when sodium is not limited.

Food	Amount	gm	Protein gm	Potassium mg	Potassium mEq	Sodium mg	Sodium mEq	Phosphorus mg	Phosphorus mEq	Calories
Bread: French, Italian, Vienna, regular	1 piece	25	2.2	22	0.6	[145]	[6.3]	21	1.2	66
Cornflakes, added nutrients	1 cup	20	1.6	14	0.4	[201]	[8.7]	9	0.5	74
Crackers, soda, unsalted tops	4 crackers	11	1.0	12	0.3	[121]	[5.3]	10	0.6	48
Farina, quick cooking, dry	2 tbsp	20	2.3	17	0.4	[50]	[2.2]	[112]	[3.6]	72

FATS AND OILS

Not an exchange list

	Portion Measure	Weight gm	Protein gm	Potassium mg	mEq	Sodium mg	mEq	Phosphorus mg	mEq	Calories
Butter or margarine, salt free	1 tbsp	14	(0)	(0)		(0)		2	0.1	100
Oils, salad or cooking; veg fats; lard	1 tbsp	14	0	0		0		0		117
Mayonnaise, prepared without salt	1 tbsp	14	—	5	0.1	0		4	0.2	101
Toppings (Whips):										
Birdseye Cool Whip (Manufacturer's data)	2 tbsp	9	0	0		2	0.1	2	0.1	32
Rich's Whip Topping (Manufacturer's data)	2 tbsp	7	0	(0)		4	0.2	(0)		20

SWEETS

List 1   Sugars, Syrups, Jellies

Exchange Value: Protein 0   Sodium 4 mg (0.2 mEq)
Potassium 7 mg (0.2 mEq)   Phosphorus 1 mg (0.1 mEq)   Calories 50

	Portion Measure	Weight gm	Protein gm	Potassium mg	mEq	Sodium mg	mEq	Phosphorus mg	mEq	Calories
Corn syrup, light or dark	1 tbsp	21	0	1	(0)	14	0.6	3	0.2	60
Jams and preserves	1 tbsp	20	0.1	18	0.5	2	0.1	2	0.1	54
Jellies	1 tbsp	18	(0)	14	0.4	3	0.1	1	0.1	49
Sugar, white, granulated	1 tbsp	11	0	0	0	(0)		(0)		42
Sugar, powdered	2 tbsp	15	0	0	0	(0)		(0)		58

Average 52

List 2   Candy and Honey

Not an exchange list

	Portion Measure	Weight gm	Protein gm	Potassium mg	mEq	Sodium mg	mEq	Phosphorus mg	mEq	Calories
Candy:										
Fondant, uncoated mints		28	0	1	(0)	[59]	[2.6]	2	0.1	102
Gumdrops		28	0	1	(0)	10	0.4	(0)	—	97
Hard sugar candy		28	0	1	(0)	9	0.4	2	0.1	108
Jelly beans		28	0	(0)		9	0.4	1	0.1	103
Marshmallows		28	0.6	2	0.1	11	0.5	2	0.1	89
Honey	1 tbsp	21	0	10	0.3	1	(0)	1	0.1	65

MISCELLANEOUS—LOW POTASSIUM

	Portion Measure	Weight gm	Protein gm	Potassium mg	mEq	Sodium mg	mEq	Phosphorus mg	mEq	Calories
Baking powder, regular, sodium al sulphate:										
With mono calcium phosphate monohydrate and calcium carbonate	1 tsp	4	0	—		[465]	[20.2]	58	3.4	3
Bouillon cubes	1 cube	4	0.8	4	0.1	[960]	[41.7]	—		5
Coca-Cola® (Manufacturer's data)	10 oz bottle	280	(0)	(0)		(0)		16	0.9	120
Kool-Aid,® sugar-sweetened soft drink mix diluted per manufacturer's directions[1]:										
Lemonade®	8 oz cup		0	1.9	(0)	19.6	0.8	19	1.1	89
Other flavors	8 oz cup		0	0.7	(0)	5.8	0.2	19	1.1	89
Kool-Aid,® instant soft drink mix, diluted per manufacturer's directions[2]:										
Lemonade and lemon-lime	8 oz cup		0	0.8	(0)	15.5	0.1	19	1.1	100
Other flavors	8 oz cup		0	0.2	(0)	16.5	0.7	19	1.1	100
Gelatin dessert base:										
D-Zerta® gelled products, clear, made with water according to manufacturer's directions:										
Orange flavor	1/2 cup	121	1.6	—		36	1.6	—		9
Other flavors	1/2 cup	121	1.6	—		30	1.3	—		8

MISCELLANEOUS—LOW POTASSIUM (Continued)

	Portion Measure	Weight gm	Protein gm	Potassium mg	Potassium mEq	Sodium mg	Sodium mEq	Phosphorus mg	Phosphorus mEq	Calories
Jello® gelled products, clear, made with water according to manufacturer's directions:										
All flavors, average value	1/2 cup	139	1.7	—		56	2.4			81
Gin, rum, vodka, or whiskey, 90 proof	1 oz	28	0	1	(0)		(0)	—		74
Ices, water, lime (no milk)	1/2 cup	100	0.4	3	0.1	(0)		(0)		78
Popsicles,® commercial[3]	One	80	—	25	0.6	140	6.0			74
Seven-UP® (Manufacturer's data):										
Regular	7 oz bottle	196	0	0		19	0.8	(0)		85
Diet	7 oz bottle	196	0	0		22	1.0	(0)		24
Salt, regular	1 packet	1	0	(0)		[388]	[16.9]	—		
Vinegar:										
Cider	1 tbsp	15	0	15	0.4	(0)		1		2
Distilled	1 tbsp	15	0	2	0.1	(0)		—		2
Water (variable, see text)										
Yeast, active, dry	1 pkg	7	2.6	140	3.6	6	0.3	90	0.3	20

[1]Composition data courtesy of General Foods Corporation.
[2]Composition data courtesy of General Foods Corporation.
[3]Sodium and potassium as analyzed in chemistry laboratories at University Hospitals, University of Wisconsin.

(1963) were markedly different from recent figures (Gormican, 1970).
3. New items appear on the market frequently and formulas are changed without notice.
4. Fluids may be restricted.

Watt and Merrill (1963) list the following values for tea and coffee in Handbook No 8:

	Potassium mg/100 gm	mEq	Sodium mg/100 gm	mEq	Phosphorus mg/100 gm	mEq
Instant coffee (dry powder)	3,256	83.5	72	3.1	383	22.2
Beverage made with instant coffee	36	0.9	1	—	4	0.2
Instant tea (dry powder)	4,530	116.0	—	—	—	—
Beverage made with instant tea	25	0.6	—	—	—	—

REFERENCES: DIET IN RENAL DISEASE

Alper, C: Fluid and electrolyte balance. In Wohl, MG; Goodhart, RS (Eds.): *Modern Nutrition in Health and Disease*. Philadelphia, Lea Febiger, 1968, Chap 12.

Anderson, FC, et al: Nutritional therapy for adults with renal disease. *JAMA, 223*:68, 1973.

Applegate, GW: Nutritional goals for dialysis patients. Unpublished paper presented at North Central Dialysis and Transplant Society, Second Annual Meeting, Univ of Wis, Madison, Wisconsin. June 16, 1972.

Avioli, LV: Intestinal absorption of calcium. *Arch Int Med, 129*:345, 1972.

———, et al: The nature of vitamin D resistance of patients with chronic renal disease. *Proc of 4th Int Congr Nephrol, 2*:175, 1970.

Berlyne, GM (Ed.): *Nutrition in Renal Disease*. Baltimore, Williams and Wilkins, 1968.

———: Medical management of chronic renal failure. *Practitioner, 201*:452, 1968.

———, et al: Low protein diet in conservative management of chronic renal failure. *Proc 4th Int Congr Nephrol, 2*:220, 1970.

———; Shaw, AB: Giordano-Giovannetti diet in terminal renal failure. *Lancet, 2*:7, 1965.

Black, DAK (Ed.): *Renal Disease*, 3rd ed. Philadelphia, Davis, 1973.

Bricker, NS: Acute renal failure. In Beeson, BP; McDermott, W (Eds.): *Cecil-Loeb Textbook of Medicine*. Philadelphia, Saunders, 1971.

California Dietetic Assoc: *A Guide to Protein Controlled Diets*. California Dietetic Assoc Central Office, 1609 Westward Blvd No 101, Los Angeles 90024.

Comty, CM: Long-term dietary management of dialysis patients. *J Am Diet Assoc, 53*:439, and 445, 1968.

Davidsohn, I; Henry, JB (Eds.): *Todd-Sanford Clinical Diagnosis by Laboratory Methods,* 14th ed. Philadelphia, Saunders, 1969.

De Luca, HF; Avioli, LV: Treatment of renal osteo-dystrophy with 25 hydroxycholecalciferol. *Arch Intern Med, 126*:896, 1970.

————: Vitamin D: A new look at an old vitamin. *Nutr Rev, 29*:179, 1971.

Dudrick, SJ; Rhoads, JE: New horizons for intravenous feeding. *JAMA, 215*:939, 1971.

Geschickter, CJ; Antonovych, TT: *The Kidney in Health and Disease.* Philadelphia, Lippincott, 1971.

Giordano, C: Use of exogenous and endogenous urea for protein synthesis in normal and uremic subjects. *J Lab Clin Med, 62*:231, 1963.

————, et al: Protein malnutrition in the treatment of chronic uremia. In Berlyne, GM (Ed.): *Nutrition in Renal Disease.* Baltimore, Williams and Wilkins, 1968.

Giovannetti, S; Maggiore, Q: A low-nitrogen diet with proteins of high biologic value for severe chronic uremia. *Lancet, 1*:1000, 1964.

Gormican, A: Inorganic elements in foods used in hospital menus. *J Am Diet Assoc, 56*:397, 1970

————: Sodium in foods and beverages. *J Milk Food Tech, 35*:1, 1972.

Gulyassy, PF, et al: Hemodialysis and plasma amino acid composition in chronic renal failure. *Am J Clin Nutr, 21*:565, 1968.

Josephson, B; Bergstrom, J, et al: Intravenous amino acid treatment in uremia. *Proc 4th Int Congr Nephrol, 2*:203, 1970.

Karp, NRS: Electrodialyzed whey based foods in chronic uremia. *J Am Diet Assoc, 59*:568, 1971.

Kerr, DNS: Chronic renal failure. In Beeson, BP; McDermott, W (Eds.): *Cecil-Loeb Textbook of Medicine.* Philadelphia, Saunders, 1971.

Kincaid-Smith, P: Treatment of irreversible renal failure by dialysis and transplantation. In Beeson, BP; McDermott, W (Eds.): *Cecil-Loeb Textbook of Medicine.* Philadelphia, Saunders, 1971.

Kopple, JD, et al: Optimal dietary protein intake during chronic hemo-dialysis. *Trans Am Soc Artif Intern Organs, 15*:302, 1969.

Krawitt, LP; Weinberger, EK: *Practical Low Protein Cookery.* Springfield, Thomas, 1971.

Lange, K: Nutritional management of kidney disorders. *Med Clin North Am, 55*:513, 1971.

Levin, S; Winklestein, JA: Diet and infrequent peritoneal dialysis. *N Engl J Med, 277*:619, 1967.

Loma Linda Medical Center Dietary Dept: *Low Protein Diets Made Simple.* Loma Linda University, Loma Linda, California 52354.

Mackenzie, JC: Nutrition and dialysis. In Bourne, GH (Ed.): *World Rev Nutr Diet, 13*:194-276, 1971.

Maddox, RK: Background and general considerations for the physician. In de St Joer, ST, et al: *Low Protein Diets for the Treatment of Chronic Renal Failure.* Salt Lake City, University of Utah Press, 1970.

Margie, JD, et al: *Mayo Clinic Renal Diet Cookbook.* New York, Western Publishing, 1973.

Mathews, DM; Laster, L: Absorption of protein digestive products. A review. *Gut, 6*:411, 1965.

Merrill, JP: Acute renal failure. In Strauss, MB; Welt, LG (Eds.): *Diseases of the Kidney,* 2nd ed. Boston, Little Brown, 1971, pp. 637-666.

Mitchell, MC; Smith, EJ: Dietary care of the patient with chronic oliguria. *Am J Clin Nutr, 19*:163, 1966.

Pearson, RE; Fish, KH: Potassium content of selected medicines, foods, and salt substitutes. *Hosp Pharmacy, 6* (no 9):6, 1971.

Phillips, S: Low protein bread. *Nutrition, 25*:93, summer, 1971.

Potassium imbalance. Programmed instruction. *Am J Nursing, 67*:343, 1967.

Recipes for Protein-Restricted Diets, 3rd ed. Minneapolis, Minnesota, Doyle Pharmaceutical Co.

Robinson, C: *Normal and Therapeutic Nutrition,* 14th ed. New York, Macmillan, 1971.

Schreiner, GS: Acute renal failure. In Black, DAK: *Renal Disease,* 3rd ed. Philadelphia, Davis, 1973.

Seldin, DW; Carter, NW; Rector, FC: Consequences of renal failure and their management. In Strauss, MB; Welt, LG (Eds.): *Diseases of the Kidney,* 2nd ed. Boston, Little Brown, 1971.

Shaw, AB, et al: Treatment of chronic renal failure by a modified Giovannetti diet. *Quart J Med, 134*:237, 1965.

Smith, EB: Gluten-free breads for patients with uremia. *J Am Diet Assoc, 59*:572, 1971.

———; Hill, PA: Protein in diets of uremic patients. *J Am Diet Assoc, 60*:389, 1972.

Sorenson, MK: A yeast leavened, low protein, low electrolyte bread. *J Am Diet Assoc, 56*:521, 1970.

Tsaltsas, TT: Dietetic management of uremic patients: Extraction of potassium from foods for uremic patients. *Am J Clin Nutr, 22*:490, 1969.

Wing, AJ: Optimum calcium concentration of dialysis fluid for maintenance haemodialysis. *Br Med J, 4*:145, Oct, 1968.

Zintel, HA: Nutrition in the care of the surgical patient. In Wohl, MG; Goodhart, RS (Eds.): *Modern Nutrition in Health and Disease,* 4th ed. Philadelphia, Lea Febiger, 1968.

INCREASED POTASSIUM IN THE DIET

Under the conditions of increased potassium losses, usually following injury, stress, gastrointestinal losses (vomiting, diarrhea, nasogastric suction without adequate parenteral replacement of

TABLE VI-6
DIET PLAN: POTASSIUM 100 mEq

Servings of foods from Table VI-5. Protein-Potassium-Sodium Exchanges, unless otherwise noted.

	Measure	Weight gm	Protein gm	Potassium mEq	Sodium mEq	Phosphorus mEq	Calories
Milk Group							
Milk, whole	2 cups	488	17.0	18.0	10.6	26.4	320
Half & half	1/2 cup	120	3.8	4.0	2.4	6.0	160
Meat, poultry, fish							
Lean products, cooked	5 exchanges	See list	40.0	13.5	5.0	20.5	275
Eggs, 3 in a week	3/7		2.6	0.7	1.1	2.6	34
Vegetables							
List 1	1 exchange	See list	1.0	4.0	0.3	1.5	20
List 2	1 exchange	See list	2.0	6.0	0.3	2.1	25
Table VI-7: potato, large, baked in skin	3/lb	150	3.9	19.3	0.3	5.7	140
Fruit							
List 3	1 exchange	See list	0.5	3.0	0.1	0.8	70
List 5	2 exchanges	See list	2.0	10.0	0.4	1.6	120
Table VI-7: 1 banana or 1/3 cup dates, or 1 cup conc pineapple juice	1 portion	See list	1.1	9.5	(0)	1.5	85
Bread-cereals							
Table VI-7: whole wheat bread (with 2% milk solids)	4 slices	100	10.4	6.8	23.2	13.2	240
Table VI-7: whole wheat cereal	2 tbsp, dry	20	2.7	1.9	0.1	4.6	68
Fats, Table VI-7							
Regular butter or margarine	1 tbsp	14	0.1	0.1	6.0	0.1	100
Regular mayonnaise	1 tbsp	14	(0)	0.1	3.6	0.2	100
Sweets, Table VI-7							
Brown sugar, firmly packed	2 tbsp	28	0	2.4	0.4	0.4	104
	Totals		87.1	99.3	53.8	87.2	1861

Regular bread, butter, and mayonnaise are included in this plan, but no salt is used in food preparation other than what is listed in the description of the foods. No salt is added at the table.

water and electrolytes) or diuretic treatment, additional potassium may be required.

An increased potassium intake may be attained either by medication or by the addition of foods relatively high in potassium to a well-selected diet. A plan for foods that provide about 100 mEq potassium is outlined in Table VI-6.

Table VI-7 lists foods that may be used in place of similar foods of lower potassium content, or may be added to the diet within calorie limits. Individual values for protein, potassium, sodium, phosphorus, and calories are given for foods in this list. Averages for foods in a group are not calculated. These foods in the quantities shown in Table VI-7 are not exchanges.

It is difficult to increase the potassium of the diet without increasing calories as well. Routine selection for a 3500 calorie diet provided 110 mEq potassium. If calorie levels are limited, a potassium supplement may be the solution.

To increase potassium beyond the 100 mEq of the basic diet plan:

1. Add more milk. Skim milk has about the same potassium content as whole milk. Cheese spread is higher in potassium than natural or processed cheeses.
2. Use more or stronger coffee, tea or decaffeinated beverage.
3. Add more fruit juices and high potassium fruits. Include at least 6 servings of vegetables and fruits per day. Dark green and leafy vegetables furnish a high ratio of potassium per 100 calories. The water in which the vegetables are cooked can be saved for making soup, hence utilizing the potassium leached during cooking. Raw vegetables will provide the most potassium.
4. Use dried fruit and nuts freely.
5. Use peanut butter as spread for bread, or add to mayonnaise for salad dressing.
6. Include baked goods made with baking powder, molasses, dried fruit, if calorie level permits.

When potassium by medication is prescribed it is desirable that the daily amount be divided into smaller quantities for distribution during the day, and that some food accompany each dose. Dilution in a suitable fluid is recommended. (Potassium supplements in tablet form, such as potassium chloride, may cause ulcerations in the gastrointestinal tract. Therefore the physician should only order potassium supplements which are in liquid form, even though there are a few such tablets still on the market).

TABLE VI-7
FOODS OF HIGHER PROTEIN AND/OR POTASSIUM VALUE

Not usually included in a protein-potassium-sodium restricted diet. When a diet is less restricted in potassium or an increased intake of potassium is desirable, selections may be made from these lists. Salt added in cooking and serving not calculated in values given. Note particularly the high potassium content of "dietetic" foods.

	Portion Measure	Portion gm	Protein gm	Potassium mg	Potassium mEq	Sodium mg	Sodium mEq	Phosphorus mg	Phosphorus mEq	Calories
Milk Group (High Potassium)										
Cheese, Cellu Low Sodium[1]		28	7.2	112	2.9	3	0.1	142	8.3	108
Cheese spread, processed American		28	4.5	67	1.7	[455]	[19.8]	245	14.2	64
Milk, 2% fat, 2% non-fat milk solids added	1 cup	246	10.0	430	11.0	150	6.5	276	16.0	145
Nuts (High Potassium)										
Almonds, dried		28	5.3	216	5.5	1	(0)	141	8.2	169
Almond meal, partially defatted		28	11.0	397	10.2	2	0.1	255	14.8	114
Cashew nuts		28	4.8	130	3.3	4	0.2	104	6.0	157
Coconut, dried, sweetened		28	1.0	99	2.5	—	—	31	1.8	153
Peanuts, roasted		28	7.3	196	5.0	1	(0)	114	6.6	163
Peanut butter, regular, added fat and sweetener	2 tbsp	28	7.1	183	4.7	[170]	[7.4]	101	5.9	163
Pecans		28	2.6	169	4.4	trace		81	4.7	192
Walnuts, English		28	4.1	126	3.2	1	(0)	106	6.2	182
Legumes (High Protein-High Potassium)										
Beans, lima, immature:										
Frozen fordhook, boiled, drained	5/8 cup	100	6.0	426	10.9	101	4.4	90	5.2	99
Frozen baby limas, boiled, drained	5/8 cup	100	7.4	394	8.9	129	5.1	126	7.3	118
Beans, lima, mature dry seeds, cooked		100	8.2	612	15.7	2	0.1	154	8.9	138
Beans, red mature, canned solids and liquid	3/8 cup	100	5.7	264	6.8	3	0.1	109	6.3	90
Beans, white, mature seeds:										
Boiled, plain	**5/8 cup**	**100**	7.8	416	10.7	7	0.3	148	8.6	118

[1]Analysis courtesy of Chicago Dietetic Supply, Inc.

Food	Measure	Weight								
Canned with pork and tomato sauce	3/8 cup	100	6.1	210	5.4	[463]	[20.0]	92	5.4	122
Lentils, mature dry seeds, cooked	1/2 cup	100	7.8	249	6.4	(0)	1.7	119	6.9	106
Peas, mature split, uncooked	1/2 cup	100	24.2	895	22.9	40		268	15.6	348
Peas, blackeye (cowpeas)										
Frozen, boiled, drained	5/8 cup	100	8.9	337	8.6	39	1.7	168	9.7	130
Canned, solids and liquid	1/2 cup	100	5.0	352	9.0	[236]	[10.3]	112	6.5	70
Vegetables (High Potassium)										
Potatoes, white:										
Baked in skin, 4 to lb	1 small	100	2.6	503	12.9	4	0.2	95	5.5	93
Baked in skin, 3 to lb	1 large	150	3.9	754	19.3	6	0.3	98	5.7	140
Boiled in skin	1 small	100	2.1	407	10.4	3	0.1	53	3.1	114
Spinach, raw, trimmed, chopped	1 cup	52	1.7	254	6.5	38	1.7	27	1.6	14
Squash, winter:										
Acorn, baked		100	1.9	480	12.3	1	(0)	29	1.7	83
Butternut, baked		100	1.1	609	15.6	1	(0)	72	4.2	80
Sweet potatoes:										
Fresh, baked	1/2 potato	100	2.1	300	7.7	12	0.5	58	3.4	141
Fresh, boiled in skin	1/2 potato	100	1.7	243	6.2	10	0.4	47	2.7	114
Canned, regular pack in syrup	1 cup	100	1.0	120	3.1	48	2.1	29	1.7	114
Yams, raw	1/2 yam	100	2.1	600	15.4	—	—	90	5.2	101
Grain Foods (High Potassium)										
Breads:										
Pumpernickel (whole rye)	1 slice	25	2.3	113	2.9	142	6.2	57	3.3	62
Raisin	1 slice	25	1.6	58	1.5	91	4.0	22	1.3	66
Whole wheat, 2% milk solids added	1 slice	25	2.6	68	1.7	133	5.8	57	3.3	60
Cereals:										
Allbran, added sugar and malt	1/3 cup	20	2.5	214	5.5	212	9.2	236	13.8	48
Bran flakes with raisins (Processor's analysis)	1/2 cup	20	2.0	106	2.7	72	3.1	63	3.7	73
Oatmeal, dry	1/4 cup	20	2.8	70	1.8	(0)		81	4.7	78
Shredded wheat without salt	3/4 biscuit	20	2.0	70	1.8	1	(0)	78	4.5	70
Wheat cereal, whole meal, dry	2 tbsp	20	2.7	74	1.9	2	0.1	81	4.7	78

	Portion		Protein	Potassium		Sodium		Phosphorus		Calories
	Measure	gm	gm	mg	mEq	mg	mEq	mg	mEq	
Wheat germ cereal	1/4 cup	28	8.4	265	6.8	30	1.3	325	18.9	109
Wheat flour, all purpose, enriched	2 tbsp	16	1.7	15	0.4	(0)		14	0.9	58
Crackers										
Graham	4 crackers	28	2.2	107	2.8	73	3.2	40	2.3	108
Rye	3 crackers	20	2.6	120	3.1	176	7.6	78	4.5	69
Macaroni, cooked until tender	1/2 cup	70	2.4	43	1.1	1	(0)	35	2.0	78
Fruits (High Potassium)										
Fresh, raw:										
Apricots	3	100	1.0	281	7.2	1	(0)	23	1.3	51
Avocado	1/2 small	100	2.1	604	15.5	4	0.2	42	2.4	167
Banana, weight without skin	1 small	100	1.1	370	9.5	1	(0)	26	1.5	85
Cantaloup or honeydew	2/3 cup	100	0.7	251	6.4	12	0.5	16	0.9	30
Nectarines		100	0.6	294	7.5	6	0.3	24	1.4	64
Plums, damson, 8 to lb	2 plums	100	0.5	299	7.7	2	0.1	17	1.0	66
Dried, uncooked										
Apricots	1/8 lb	57	0.6	558	14.3	15	0.7	62	3.6	148
Dates	1/8 lb	57	1.3	370	9.5	1	(0)	36	2.1	156
Figs	1/8 lb	57	2.5	365	9.3	1	(0)	44	2.5	156
Peaches	1/8 lb	57	1.8	542	14.0	9	0.4	67	3.9	149
Pears	1/8 lb	57	1.8	327	8.4	4	0.2	27	1.6	153
Prunes, "softenized"	1/8 lb	57	1.2	395	10.1	5	0.2	45	2.6	145
Raisins	1/8 lb	57	1.4	435	11.2	15	0.7	58	3.4	165
Juices										
Apple juice	1 cup	248	0.2	250	6.4	2	0.1	22	1.3	120
Apricot nectar	1 cup	251	0.7	378	9.7	(0)		30	1.8	140
Grapefruit juice, canned	1 cup	247	1.2	400	10.3	2	0.1	35	2.0	165
Grapefruit juice, conc, unsweetened frozen, diluted 1 to 3	1 cup	247	1.2	420	10.8	2	0.1	42	2.4	100
Grapefruit juice, orange juice blended, frozen concentrate diluted 1 to 3	1 cup	250	1.5	443	11.4	(0)		33	1.9	110

Grape juice, canned or bottled	1 cup	253	0.5	293	7.5	5	0.2	30	1.8	165
Orange juice, conc, frozen diluted 1 to 3	1 cup	249	1.8	467	12.0	2	0.1	40	2.3	120
Orange-apricot drink, canned	1 cup	249	0.5	235	6.0	(0)		20	1.2	125
Pineapple juice, canned, unsweetened	1 cup	249	1.0	371	9.5	2	0.1	22	1.3	135
Prune juice, canned or bottled	1 cup	256	1.0	602	15.4	4	0.2	52	3.0	200
Sweets, (High Potassium)										
Cane syrup	1 tbsp	20	—	85	2.2	—		—		53
Maple syrup	1 tbsp	20	—	35	0.9	2	0.1	2	0.1	50
Molasses, light	1 tbsp	20	—	183	4.7	3	0.1	9	0.5	50
Molasses, medium	1 tbsp	20	—	213	5.5	7	0.3	14	0.8	46
Sugar, brown	1 tbsp	14	—	48	1.2	4	0.2	4	0.2	52
Fats, Regular (High Sodium)										
Butter or margarine	1 tbsp	14	0.1	3	0.1	138	6.0	2	0.1	100
French dressing	1 tbsp	16	0	12	0.3	206	9.0	2	0.1	65
Mayonnaise	1 tbsp	14	(0)	5	0.1	83	3.6	4	0.2	100
Beverages, Beverage Components and Broth (High Potassium)										
Beer	1 cup	240	0.7	60	1.5	17	0.7	7	0.4	101
Broth, beef, condensed, canned, diluted 1 to 1[1]		100	1.8	45	1.2	[354]	[15.4]	(0)		18
Broth, chicken, condensed, canned, diluted 1 to 1[1]		100	2.8	85	2.2	[393]	[17.1]	30	1.8	18
Chocolate, bitter	1 oz	28	3.0	232	6.0	1	(0)	124	7.2	141
Chocolate syrup, thin type	1 tsp	15	0.3	42	1.1	8	0.3	14	0.8	36
Chocolate mix for hot chocolate, dry	1 packet	28	2.6	169	4.3	[107]	[4.7]	81	4.7	110
Cocoa, dry powder	1 tsp	2	(0)	30	0.8	(0)		13	0.8	5
Cocoa powder with non-fat milk	2 tbsp	28	5.0	224	5.7	[147]	[6.4]	153	8.9	146
Coffee, instant dry powder	1 tsp	1	0	33	0.8	1	(0)	(0)		(0)
Coffee, brewed from grounds (Gormican, 1970)	8 oz cup	240	0	156	4.0	2	0.1	8	0.5	(0)
Consomme, chicken, condensed, canned, diluted 1 to 1[2]		100	1.5	30	0.8	[325]	[14.1]	16	0.9	9

	Portion		Protein	Potassium		Sodium		Phosphorus		Calories
	Measure	gm	gm	mg	mEq	mg	mEq	mg	mEq	
Tea, steeped (Gormican, 1970)	8 oz cup	240	0	22	0.6	2	0.1	1	0.1	(0)
Wine, dessert	1/3 cup	70	0	53	1.4	3	0.1	—		96
Wine, table	1/3 cup	70	0	64	1.6	4	0.2	7	0.4	60
Food Adjuncts (High Potassium)										
Baking powder, "dietetic" low sodium, commercial	1 tsp	4	0	438	11.2	(0)		292	17.0	7
Catsup	1 tbsp	15	0.3	54	1.4	[154]	[6.7]	8	0.5	19
Salt substitutes:										
Adolph's Dietetic Salt Substitute[3]	1 packet	1	0	430	11.2	0		—		
Cosalt[4]		1	0	450	11.5	0		—		
Diasal[4]		1	0	442	11.3	0		—		
Neocurtasal[4]		1	0	470	12.1	0		—		
Soy sauce		10	0.6	36	0.9	[732]	[32.0]	10	0.6	
Garlic cloves		1	—	5	0.1	—		2	0.1	
Gelatin, plain	1 tbsp	7	6	—		1.4	0.6	—		23

[1]Data courtesy of Campbell Soup Company.
[2]Data courtesy of Heinz Company.
[3]Data courtesy of Adolph's Ltd, Burbank, California.
[4]Pearson and Fish: *Hospital Pharmacy, 6* (no 9), 1971.

RESTRICTED PHENYLALANINE DIET

Phenylketonuria is an inherited inborn error of metabolism; the amino acid, phenylalanine, cannot be metabolized in the normal manner. Lack of proper mental development may result from either a deficiency or an excess of phenylalanine under such conditions.

A modified formula low in phenylalanine is used to provide the phenylketonuric (PKU) neonate's recommended daily allowance of protein. Other natural foods containing protein are carefully selected to provide sufficient phenylalanine for normal growth (200 to 325 mg per day during first three years of life) while avoiding either a deficiency or an excess (Berry, Hunt, Sutherland 1971). The restricted phenylalanine diet is used exclusively for the treatment of infants and children with phenylketonuria.

Diet Plan

A low phenylalanine formula is the major source of nourishment for patients receiving the restricted phenylalanine diet. The low phenylalanine formula most commonly used in the United States is Lofenalac because of its nutrient supplementation and its wide acceptance. Other products are available, and more are being developed. Some products which appear to have considerable value are being used in Great Britain and are being tested (1973) for acceptance by the Food and Drug Administration for distribution in the United States.

Each of the low phenylalanine products on the market has its own composition and cannot be interchanged with another without further dietary calculation. Only Lofenalac will be discussed here. It is fortified with vitamins and minerals in amounts comparable to the usual cow's milk formula. It contains supplementary vitamin C. It provides 15 percent of its calories as protein, 35 percent as fat, and 50 percent as carbohydrate. Mixed in a normal dilution (1 to 4) Lofenalac provides 20 calories per ounce. See Table VI-10 for calories, protein and phenylalanine content at 3 different dilutions.

Berry, Hunt and Sutherland (1971) recommended following the NAS-NRC Recommended Dietary Allowances in calculating calorie and protein levels for the PKU child. Based on Holt and Snyderman's (1967) amino acid study, they allow 70 to 90 mg phenylalanine per kg body weight for children up to 2 years of age. From

2 to 10 years they allow 30 mg phenylalanine per kg, decreasing to 25 mg at 10 years, the latter being the level recommended by Nagagawa et al (1962) for 10 year olds.

Smith and Waisman (1971) recommended a phenylalanine intake of 60 mg per kg body weight for the PKU infant, the same as for the normal infant. Berry, et al consider a plasma phenylalanine level of 5 to 10 mg per 100 milliliters to be optimum for growth and development.

Berry, Hunt, and Sutherland (1971) prescribe sufficient Lofenalac formula to meet the infant's protein allowance. Lofenalac, dry, provides 1.4 gms protein per tablespoon. The phenylalanine in this amount of Lofenalac (7.5 mg phenylalanine per tablespoon dry weight, 43 calories) is subtracted from the calculated phenylalanine need (70 to 90 mg per kg body weight) to find how much additional phenylalanine is needed. This amount is then furnished in natural (or "supplemental") foods including limited quantities of milk.

For the different age groups, Berry et al have provided tables with these calculations and additional data to assist in adjusting food patterns as the child grows. Lofenalac feedings should always be accompanied by supplemental foods to provide a balanced amino acid intake. Limited quantities of regular protein foods are introduced as the child grows older.

Plasma prenylalanine levels *and* growth rates determine when additional phenylalanine is needed. Generally the phenylalanine needs will fall within the ranges discussed above. Additional calories must be provided as needed for normal growth. The other objectives of the diet will be the same as for any pediatric diet.

A phenylalanine exchange system is commonly used for restricted phenylalanine diets for children. In the amounts listed, each food will provide approximately 15 mg phenylalanine and may be exchanged for any other serving of food on the list. The following is adapted from a list prepared by Smith and Swanson in 1971. It must be emphasized that food processors' formulas change without notice, so these values should be checked. They are set up to allow flexibility of selection within food groups. However, if all foods within a basic group are refused, it is important to replace from another group rather than allow the child to be under his phenylalanine quota for the day.

See Appendix IV for references on the amino acid content of foods and for commercial sources of dietary products and technical information on special ingredients. Cost will be lower if natural foodstuffs are used. No special products other than the low phenylalanine milk are recommended.

The following objectives must be met for the phenylketonuric child:

1. Use Lofenalac or similar low phenylalanine product, as the source of nourishment.
2. Supply additional phenylalanine needed as determined by plasma phenylalanine determinations *and* by growth rates. Generally the phenylalanine needs will fall within the ranges discussed above.
3. Provide additional calories as needed for normal growth. Growth rate should be normal.
4. Other objectives will be the same as for any pediatric diet.

TABLE VI-8
CALORIE, PROTEIN, AND PHENYLALANINE CONTENT OF LOFENALAC AT THREE DIFFERENT DILUTIONS

This table is useful when the amount of protein in the diet needs to be increased as the child becomes older. If the child will not take the larger volume of liquid, select the higher concentration for use at any age.

Lofenalac Powder (packed)	Volume	Calories	Protein gm	Phenylalanine mg
1 scoop = 1 tablespoon	1 scoop	42.5	1.41	7.5
1 8-ounce measuring cup level (150 gm)	1 cup	680	22.5	120
Dilution:	*Volume After*			
Lofenalac Powder to Water	*Dilution*			
Normal dilution: 1 to 4 by volume	1 ounce	19.3	0.64	3.4
	8 ounces	154	5.1	27
	24 ounces	463	15.4	82
1½ strength: 1 to 3 by volume	1 ounce	25	0.83	4.4
	8 ounces	200	6.6	35
	24 ounces	600	19.9	106
Double strength: 1 to 2 by volume	1 ounce	35.4	1.17	6.2
	8 ounces	283	9.4	50
	24 ounces	850	28.1	149

TABLE VI-9
PHENYLALANINE EXCHANGE LIST

Adapted from lists developed by Barbara Johnson Smith and Marilyn Ribbe Swanson, University of Wisconsin Center for Health Sciences

FRUIT

Amount containing one (1)

Food	Phenylalanine Exchange (15 mg)	Reference*
(all canned fruit in medium syrup; served with 2 tbsp syrup)		
Apples (about 3/lb; 2-1/2 in diam)	2 medium	AW
Applesauce, canned	1 cup	AW

Food	Amount containing one (1) Phenylalanine Exchange (15 mg)	Reference*
Apricots, dried	2 halves	AW
Apricots, canned	2 halves	AW
Avocado	1/3 cup	AW
Banana, medium (9 x 1-1/2 in)	1/3 banana (3 tbsp mashed)	AW
Blackberries, raw or canned	1/3 cup	AW
Blueberries, raw or frozen	10 tbsp	AW
Cantaloup (medium, 5 in diam)	1/6 melon (or 1/2 cup diced)	MOW
Cherries, sweet or sour	1/2 cup	AW
Cranberries, raw or cooked with sugar	1 cup	AW
Dates	2 tbsp, 2-1/2 medium dates	AW
Figs, dried	1 small fig	AW
Fruit cocktail, canned	3/4 cup	AW
Grapes	1/2 cup	AW
	1/2 medium	AW
Grapefruit, fresh	1/2 medium	AW
Grapefruit, canned	1/2 cup	MOW
Lemon	Free in moderate amounts	
Lime	Free in moderate amounts	
Muskmelon (medium, 5 in diam)	1/6 melon or 1/2 cup diced	MOW
Nectarine	1-1/2 medium	AW
Oranges (3 in diam)	1 medium, 2/3 cup sections	AW
Peaches, raw, whole (about 4/lb, 2 in diam)	1-1/2 medium or 3/4 cup slices	MOW
Peaches, canned	3/4 cup slices or 3 halves	MOW
Pears, raw (3 x 2-1/2 in)	1 pear	MOW
Pears, canned	1 cup slices or 5 halves	MOW
Pineapple, raw, diced	1 cup	Pa, AW
Pineapple, canned	3/4 cup crushed, 2 large slices	AW
Plums, raw	2 medium	AW
Plums, canned	4 medium	AW
Prunes (67/lb)	2 medium	MOW
Raisins, dried	2 tbsp	AW
Raspberries, raw or canned	1/3 cup	AW
Strawberries, raw	2/3 cup	MOW
Strawberries, frozen, sweetened	1/4 cup	AW
Tangerine	1-1/2 large, 3 small	AW
Watermelon	1/2 cup cubes	AW

FRUIT JUICE

Food	Amount	Reference
Apple juice	16 oz	(3 percent of protein)
Apricot nectar	6 oz	AW
Cranberry juice cocktail	12 oz	AW
Grapefruit juice	4 oz	AW
Grape juice	4 oz	AW
Lemondae	16 oz	(3 percent of protein)
Limeade	16 oz	(3 percent of protein)

Food	Amount containing one (1) Phenylalanine Exchange (15 mg)	Reference*
Orange juice	6 oz	AW
Peach nectar	5 oz	AW
Pineapple juice	6 oz	AW
Prune juice	4 oz	AW

VEGETABLES

Food	Amount	Reference
Asparagus, froz cuts & tips	2 tbsp, cooked	MOW
Beans, snap, raw	3 tbsp, cooked	MOW
Beans, snap, canned or frozen	3 tbsp	MOW
Beets, fresh or canned	1/2 cup, cooked	MOW
Beet greens	1 tbsp, cooked	Pa
Broccoli, frozen	1 oz, 3 tbsp	MOW
Brussels sprouts (24 sprouts/lb)	1/2 sprout, cooked	MOW
Cabbage, common varieties and chinese	1/2 cup raw	MOW
Cabbage, red and savoy	1/4 cup raw	MOW
Carrots, raw	1 carrot, 5-1/2 x 1 in	MOW
Carrots, cooked	1/3 cup	MOW
Cauliflower	3 tbsp, raw or cooked	AW
Celery, raw	1/4 cup diced	Pa
Celery, cooked	1/4 cup	AW
Chard, collards, leaves	1-1/2 tbsp cooked	AW
Corn, canned whole kernel	2 *tsp*	MOW
Cucumber, peeled	1 medium, 6" long, 2" diam	AW
Eggplant	2 tbsp, cooked	MOW
Kale	2 tbsp, cooked	AW
Kohlrabi	1/4 cup cooked or raw	MOW
Lettuce	2 large or 4 small leaves	MOW
Mustard greens	2 tbsp cooked	Pa
Okra (3 in long)	2 pods, cooked	AW
Onions	1/4 cup raw or cooked	MOW
Parsley	3 tbsp	AW
Parsnips	3 tbsp, cooked	AW
Peas, green, canned or frozen	2 *tsp,* cooked, drained	MOW
Peppers, sweet green (6 medium/lb)	1/2 medium, raw or cooked	MOW
Pickles (cucumber) sweet or dil.	3/4 cup	Pa
Pickle relish	3/4 cup	AW
Popcorn, popped	3 tbsp	AW
Potatoes, french fries (2 x 1/2 x 1/2 in)	1-1/2 pieces	AW
Potatoes, peeled, boiled	1-1/2 tbsp	AW
Potato chips (2 in diam)	3 pieces	AW
Pumpkin, canned	1/4 cup	MOW
Radish, red (1 in diam)	4 small	AW
Sauerkraut	1/2 cup	AW
Spinach	2 tbsp raw 1 tbsp cooked, drained	MOW
Squash, summer	5 tbsp cooked	Pa
Squash, winter	2 tbsp cooked	Pa
Sweet potatoes, peeled, boiled, baked or canned	1 tbsp	MOW
Tomatoes, ripe, raw	1/3 medium, 3/lb or	

Food	Amount containing one (1) Phenylalanine Exchange (15 mg)	Reference*
	1/4 cup canned solids and liquids	MOW
Tomato juice	1/4 cup	AW
Catsup	2 tbsp	AW
Turnip greens, leaves including stems	3 tbsp raw, 1-1/2 tbsp cooked	MOW
Turnips	1/2 cup raw or cooked	MOW

CEREALS AND BREADS

Bread

Resource Mix Bread	1-1/2 slices	Mfg
Wheat starch bread (special recipe)	3 slices	Mfg
White bread, no milk	1/8 slice	(5 percent of protein)

Cereal, Cooked (in water)

Cream of wheat	1 tbsp	AW
Oatmeal	1 tbsp	AW
Pablum barley cereal	1 tbsp	AW

Cereal, Ready-to-eat

Applejacks, Kellogg	3-1/2 tbsp	Pa
Captain Crunch, Quaker	3-1/2 tbsp	Pa
Cheerios	1-1/2 tbsp	Pa
Corn flakes	2-1/2 tbsp	Pa
Kix	2-1/2 tbsp	Pa
Puffed rice	5 tbsp	Pa
Rice Krispies	3 tbsp	Pa
Sugar Pops	5 tbsp	Pa
Wheaties	5 tbsp	Pa

Cookies

Fig Newton, 31/lb	2/3	Pa
Lemon Snaps (small—120/lb)	1	Pa
Lorna Doone Shortbread	1/2	Pa
Nabisco Sugar Wafers (small—148/lb)	2	Pa

Crackers

Animal cracker	2-1/2	AW
Arrowroot cookies	3/4	AW
Graham cracker	1/2 square	AW
Oyster crackers (650/lb)	5	Pa
Ritz crackers	1	AW
Saltines (2 in square)	2	AW
Tortilla, corn (6" diam)	1/4	AW
Triscuit wafer, National Biscuit	2/3	Pa
Wheat Thins	2-1/2	AW

SOUPS AND BOUILLON

Asparagus, cream of, Campbell	1-1/2 tbsp condensed	AW
Beef broth, Campbell	1 tbsp condensed	AW
Celery, Campbell	1-1/2 tbsp condensed	AW
Minestrone, Campbell	1/2 tbsp condensed	AW
Mushroom, cream of, Campbell	1 tbsp condensed	AW

Food	Amount containing one (1) Phenylalanine Exchange (15 mg)	Reference*
Onion, Campbell	1 tbsp condensed	Pa
Potato, cream of, Campbell Frozen	2-1/2 tbsp condensed	Pa
Tomato, Campbell	1 tbsp condensed	AW
Vegetarian vegetable, Campbell	1 tbsp condensed	AW

FATS AND OILS

Butter	3 tbsp	Pa
French dressing, commercial	6 tbsp	Pa
Margarine	3 tbsp	Pa
Miracle Whip	1-1/2 tbsp	Pa
Mayonnaise	1-1/2 tbsp	Pa
Shortening, vegetable	1-1/2 tbsp	Pa

(Oil is phenylalanine free, but intentional additives or the casein not completely removed from butter contribute phenylalanine.)

MISCELLANEOUS

Evaporated milk	1 tsp	(5 percent of protein)
Homogenized milk	2 tsp	(5 percent of protein)
Macaroni	1 tbsp cooked tender	(5 percent of protein)
Marshmallow	1-1/2 marshmallows, average size	(5 percent of protein)
Mustard, prepared	1 tsp	AW
Rice, brown or white	1-1/2 tbsp, cooked	AW
Spaghetti	1 tbsp cooked	AW

BABY FOODS

Quantities derived from data by McCarthy, Orr and Watt*

Amount containing one (1) Phenylalanine Exchange (15 mg)

Fruits	Junior (7-3/4 oz jar)	Strained (4-3/4 oz jar)
Applesauce	1 jar	2 jars
Peaches	1/2 jar	1 jar
Pears	3/4 jar	1-1/2 jars
Pears and Pineapple	3/4 jar	1-1/2 jars
Prunes with Tapioca	2/3 jar	2 jars
Vegetables		
Beans, snap	2 tbsp	2 tbsp
Beets	—	1/2 jar
Carrots	1/2 7-1/2 oz jar	3/4 4-3/4 oz jar
Corn, creamed	3-1/2 tbsp	2-1/2 tbsp
Squash	3 tbsp	4 tbsp
Sweet potato	2 tbsp	1-1/2 tbsp

Note: If amino acid composition is unavailable, phenylalanine content can be estimated as:
5 percent of the protein composition of animal foods, legumes, nuts and cereals.
4 percent of the protein of dark green leafy vegetables.
3 percent of the protein of other fruits and vegetables.

For fabricated and combined foods, check *recent* composition data.

Key to References Listed in Table*

AW   Acosta, PB; Wenz, E: Nutrition in phenylketonuria. In Bickel, H, et al: *Phenylketonuria and Some Inborn Errors of Amino Acid Metabolism.* Stuttgart, George Theime Verlag, 1971.

MOW McCarthy, MA; Orr, ML; Watt, BK: Phenylalanine and tyrosine in vegetables and fruits. *J Am Diet Assoc, 52*:130, 1968.

Pa   Collins, P, et al: *Pennsylvania's Guide for Diets Restricted in Phenylalanine.* Pennsylvania Department of Health, Division of Nutrition, Harrisburg, Pennsylvania, 1971.

TABLE VI-10a PROTEIN-FREE FOODS

These foods may be used freely, except as appetite for Lofenalac formula or other prescribed foods may be affected.

Beverages
> Carbonated beverages
> Koolaid
> Strawberry Quik
> Tang
> Tea

Candy
> Butterscotch candy
> Corn candy
> Fondant, patties or mints
> Gum drops
> Hard candy
> Jelly beans
> Lollipops

Fats and Oils
> Corn oil margarines that do not contain caseinate.
>> Read ingredients on label.
> Crisco
> Lard
> Salad and cooking oils—corn, olive, peanut oils, etc.

Raw Ingredients and Thickening Agents
> Baking powder
> Baking soda
> Cellu wheat starch
> Corn starch
> Flavorings: e.g. vanilla, almond, etc.
> Paygel-P wheat starch
> Tapioca, granulated
> Vinegar

Spices, Dressings, and Garnishes

Colored sugars	Parsley
Cranberry sauce or cranberry jelly	Pepper
Lemon juice or lime juice	Pickles—sweet or dill and pickle relish
Lemon or lime wedge	Salt
Maraschino cherries	Soy sauce
Mint leaf	Spices—any kind
Italian salad dressing	Vinegar and oil dressing

Sweets other than Candy

Apple butter	Molasses
Chewing gum	Popsicles
"Danish Dessert" pudding	Rich's Whip Topping or Kohl's*
made by Junket Co.	"Sherbet Mix" put out by
Honey	Junket Co., made with water
Jam	Sugar, any kind
Jelly, any kind	Syrup, any kind
Jell-Quik,	
Loma Linda Food Company	

*Read list of ingredients to make certain product does not contain *sodium caseinate.*

TABLE 10b FOODS TO AVOID

Each serving is VERY high in phenylalanine and may not be used, *even in VERY small portions,* without specific permission or recommendation of the physician or dietitian in charge of the dietary treatment.

Dairy products
    Cheese, all kinds
    Cream, all kinds
    Ice cream, ice milk, or sherbet
    Milk, all kinds
    Yogurt
Eggs
Flour, all kinds
Legumes (dried peas, dried beans, lima beans and seeds)
Meat, poultry, fish
Nuts
Peanut butter
Vegetable substitutes imitating meat, poultry, etc.

REFERENCES

Acosta, PB, et al: *PKU: A Diet Guide,* revised. Los Angeles, Children's Hospital of Los Angeles, PKU Section, 1969.

Acosta, PB; Wenz, E: Nutrition in phenylketonuria. In Bickel, H, et al: *Phenylketonuria and Some Inborn Errors of Amino Acid Metabolism.* Stuttgart: George Theime Verlag, 1971.

Ampola, MG: Phenylketonuria and other disorders of amino acid metabolism. *Pediatr Clin North Am, 20:*507, 1973.

Bertavin, A, et al: Use of an amino acid mixture in the treatment of phenylketonuria. *Arch Dis Child, 45:*640, 1970.

Berry, HK; Hunt, MM; Sutherland, BK: Amino acid balance in the treatment of phenylketonuria. *J Am Diet Assoc, 58:*210, 1971.

Block, RJ; Weiss, KW: *Amino Acid Handbook.* Springfield, Thomas, 1956.

Brooks, PV; Rogers, PJ: Low protein, low phenylalanine cakes. *J Am Diet Assoc, 54:*495, 1969.

Childrens Bureau: *Phenylketonuria: A Comprehensive Bibliography, 1964.* Childrens Bureau Publication no 430, 1966. Washington, DC, US Dept of Health, Education and Welfare, 1966.

Church, CF; Church, HN: *Food Values of Portions Commonly Used,* 11th ed. Philadelphia, Lippincott, 1970.

Francis, DEM; Dixon, DJW: *Diets for Sick Children,* 2nd ed. Oxford and Edinburgh, Blackwell Scientific Pub, 1970. (Presents the British method of treatment and describes some of their special food products. Diets for other errors in metabolism also included.)

Holt, LE, Jr; Snyderman, SE: Amino acid requirements in children. In Nyhan, WL (Ed.): *Amino Acid Metabolism and Genetic Variation.* New York, McGraw Hill, 1967, Chap 26.

Hsia, DYY: Phenylketonuria and its variants. In Steinberg, A (Ed.): *Progress in Medical Genetics,* vol 6. New York, Grune & Stratton, 1969.

Hunt, MM; Sutherland, BS; and Berry, HK: Nutritional management in phenylketonuria. *Am J Dis Child, 122*:1, 1971.

Koch, R, et al: An approach to management of phenylketonuria. *J Pediat, 76*:815, 1970.

McCarthy, MA; Orr, ML; Watt, BK: Phenylalanine and tyrosine in vegetables and fruits. *J Am Diet Assoc, 52*:130, 1968.

Miller, GT; Williams, VR; Moschette, DS: Phenylalanine content of fruit. *J Am Diet Assoc, 46*:43, 1965.

Nakagawa, I, et al: Amino acid requirements of children: Minimal needs for threonine, valine, and phenylalanine based on nitrogen balance method. *J Nutr, 77*:61, 1962.

Nutritional Values of Gerber Baby Foods. Fremont, Michigan, Gerber Products Co, 1966.

Orr, ML; Watt, BK: *Amino Acid Content of Foods.* Home Economics Research Report No 4, Household Economics Research Division, Institute of Home Economics, Agricultural Research Service, US Department of Agriculture, Washington, DC, 1957.

Robinson, CH: *Normal and Therapeutic Nutrition,* 14th ed. New York, Macmillan, 1972. (Chap 48 gives exchanges in 15 and 30 mg phenylalanine portions. Other inborn errors discussed and references given.)

Smith, BJ; Waisman, HA: Adequate phenylalanine intake for optimum growth and development in the treatment of phenylketonuria. *Am J Clin Nutr, 24*:423, 1971.

Umbarger, BJ: *Phenylalanine Content of Foods.* Cincinnati, The Children's Hospital Research Foundation, 1965.

————; Berry, HK; Sutherland, BS: Advances in the management of patients with phenylketonuria. *JAMA, 193*:784, 1965.

Wong, PW; Hsia, DY: Inborn errors of metabolism. In Goodhart, RS; Shils, ME (Eds.): *Modern Nutrition in Health and Disease,* 5th ed. Philadelphia, Lea Febiger, 1973, Chap 39.

See also references for amino acids in Appendix Four.

RESTRICTED GLUTEN DIET

Rationale

Non-tropical sprue (adult celiac disease) is a malabsorption syndrome characterized by a primary idiopathic steatorrhea which responds to a gluten-free diet. Tissue samples of the intestinal mucosa show an absence of the normal villus pattern. The extent of the secretory and absorptive changes depends upon the condition of the mucosa.

Impairment in fat absorption is common. Impaired digestion and absorption of disaccharides can occur. This is noted most frequently as a lactase deficiency (Peternel, 1968).

Children treated with a gluten-free diet generally achieve a tolerance for gluten and remain asymptomatic. However, Sheldon (1969) points out that malabsorption symptoms are likely to occur in later life. An anemia, accompanied by low serum folic acid levels may also develop. Pregnancy, infections, psychological upsets, or overindulgence may cause a relapse. For this reason Sheldon recommends that persons with this disorder remain on a gluten-free diet throughout life. Although the individual may tolerate a limited amount of gluten for extended periods, Sheldon feels that gluten in the diet increases the probability of a relapse. Poor absorption as well as elimination of most cereal products from the diet may lead to low blood levels of many minerals and vitamins particularly iron, magnesium and B vitamins. See Table I-3, page 25. Pharmaceutical supplements may be needed.

Diet Plan

Wheat, rye, oats, barley, and all foods combined with any of these grains are eliminated in this diet. Fats and oils are used in limited amounts, and foods with a high amount of fat are not included.

Milk group: The quantity appropriate to the individual is included in the diet. See the daily food guide. If the physician orders lactose restriction milk is not allowed but aged cheese (which has only a trace of lactose) may be tolerated after symptoms have abated. See lactose-restricted diet in Section VI.

Meat group: Select meats from the Lean Meat Exchange list to avoid excess fat. Avoid adding fat or wheat, oats, rice or barley products in cooking. The quantity of meat, fish or poultry may need to be increased to meet caloric needs.

Dry beans, peas, nuts: Dry beans, peas, and lentils are low in fat and may be used to advantage. Nuts are high in fat and are usually not included, but peanut butter may be used in limited amounts. If lactose is restricted, the peanut butter must be lactose-free.

Fruit and vegetables: There is no restriction for this group. Quantities may need to be increased to meet caloric needs. Note that avocados and olives have high fat content. If used, limit the quantity.

Grain foods: Cornmeal, cornstarch, tapioca and rice may be used. Instead of foods prepared with wheat, rye, oats, or barley, a special gluten-free wheat starch may be used to make breads and other baked items. Because the texture and flavor of these products are different they are generally not well received. Gluten-free wheat starch is expensive.

Fats and oils: Limited in quantity as long as symptoms persist. Avoid fried foods and commercial dressings which may contain wheat starch. Butter and margarine contain small amounts of lactose but are generally included in the maintenance diets. See restricted lactose diets.

Sugars and syrups: Limited in amount. Their best use is in combination with other foods and distributed among the day's meals.

The diet as outlined may be adapted for children by making the appropriate changes in the amounts of foods recommended. Recipes which are helpful in making the diet more palatable are provided by the companies selling wheatstarch and by Wood (1967), and Sheedy and Keifitz (1969). Addresses of some commercial sources for wheat starch are with the general references in Appendix IV.

REFERENCES

Cooke, WT: Adult celiac disease. *Prog Gastroenterol, 1*:299, 1968.
Gardner, JD; Brown, MS; Laster, L: The columnar epithelial cell of the small intestine: Digestion and transport. *New Engl J Med, 283*:1317, 1970.
Kowlessar, OD, et al: Celiac disease: Enzyme defect or immune mechanism? *Prog Gastroenterol, 2*:23, 1970.
Peternel, WW: Disaccharidase deficiency. *Med Clin N Am, 52*:1355, 1968.

Ross, JR, et al: Gluten enteropathy and skeletal disease. *JAMA, 196*:180, 1966.

Rubin, W: Celiac disease. *Am J Clin Nutr, 24*:91, 1971.

Sheedy, CM; Keifitz, N: *Cooking for Your Celiac Child.* New York, Dial Press, 1969.

Sheldon, W: Prognosis in early adult life of coeliac children treated with gluten-free diet. *Brit Med J, 2*:401, 1969.

Sleisinger, MH; Rynberger, HJ; Pert, JH; Almy, TP: A wheat-, rye-, and oat-free diet. *J Am Diet Assoc, 33*:1137, 1957.

—————: Diseases of malabsorption. In Beeson, PB; McDermott, W (Eds.): *Cecil-Loeb Textbook of Medicine,* 13th ed. Philadelphia, Saunders, 1971.

Editorial: Seeking the causes of malabsorption. *New Engl J Med, 283*: 1340, 1970.

Wood, MN: *Gourmet Food on a Wheat-Free Diet.* Springfield, Thomas, 1967. (Recipes for wheat, rye, barley and oat-free foods.)

RESTRICTED PURINE DIET

Gout is a disease associated with an increased level of uric acid in the blood. Normal serum values for uric acid vary from 2 to 5 mg per 100 ml of plasma or serum. Persons with gout have levels of 6 to 10 mg and rarely up to 20 mg per 100 ml of serum or plasma (Bayles, 1968). Primary gout is a genetically-transmitted disease; secondary gout may occur in certain other diseases or due to drug therapy.

Acute symptoms of gout are brought about by increments to deposits of monosodium urate in and about the joints. Fasting and excesses of alcohol both lead to appreciable elevations in serum urate concentration.

Since less than half of the uric acid found in the blood can be attributed to dietary components, treatment of gout relies primarily on drug therapy directed toward increasing excretion of uric acid. When symptoms of gout are severe, dietary treatment in addition to drug therapy may assist in lowering uric acid in the blood. Objectives of dietary treatment in general are:

1. Provide a diet that is adequate in essential nutrients and suitable to the caloric needs of the individual. If overweight, institute a program of moderate calorie restriction rather than drastic reduction. Avoid fasting. Severe calorie limitation may cause a rise in blood uric acid resulting in an acute attack.

2. Exclude foods particularly high in purines, and emphasize foods of negligible purine content. See lists of foods grouped according to milligrams of purine nitrogen in 100 gm in this section.

3. Limit fat consumption to not over 50 to 60 grams per day. A high level of fat in the diet limits renal excretion of uric acid.

4. Increase fluid intake. Large quantities of fluids will promote excretion of uric acid and minimize uric acid precipitation in the urinary tract.

A person who has suffered an acute attack of gouty arthritis, or whose genetic background includes gout, is well-advised to avoid foods of high purine content throughout life. During an acute attack foods may be limited to those of little or no purine content in simple, easily-digested forms. Calories adequate for maintenance should be provided, and fluids stressed.

A restricted purine diet, based on the daily food guide, may be used in the periods between acute attacks. It includes the following:

Milk: 3 to 4 cups of skim milk per day. Cheeses may be used within fat and calorie limits. Low-fat cottage cheese contains about 2% fat.

Meat, fish: Not over 3 ounces (cooked weight) per day of those that have moderate purine content. See lists of purine content of foods. Avoid broth soups, gravies, bouillon cubes, and soup bases.

Eggs: Egg yolks are limited to 3 a week. Although free of purine they have a high cholesterol content. Egg whites may be used freely.

Nuts: Limited only by the level of fat and calorie allowances.

Fruits and vegetables: May be used freely. At least four servings should be used daily including good sources of vitamins A and C.

Grain foods: White enriched bread and cereal products may be used as desired to meet caloric needs. Whole grain products should be used sparingly during an acute attack.

Fats: The limitation on the amount of fat in the diet places increased emphasis on selection of fats of good values in vitamin E (vegetable oils) and vitamin A (butter and margarine).

Sweets: Sugar, jellies, fruit preserves, and syrups may be used as desired within calorie limits.

Beverages: Coffee, tea, cocoa, Sanka, and Postum are included in the diet. An excess of alcoholic beverages should be avoided, although moderate amounts may be used at the physician's direction. Macklachlan and Rodnan (1967) found that a combination of alcohol and fasting precipitated an attack.

Purine Content of Foods

Negligible Purine Content: From 0 to 5 mg purine nitrogen in 100 gm

Milk, cheese, cottage cheese	Vegetables except as noted below.
Eggs	Enriched refined cereals and breads
Nuts, peanut butter	Oils and fats, butter, margarine
All fruits	Sugar, syrups, fruit preserves
Gelatin, tapioca, cornstarch	

Low Purine Content: From 8 to 27 mg purine nitrogen in 100 gm or 24 to 81 mg/100 gm when calculated as uric acid

Asparagus	Mushrooms
Cauliflower	Spinach

Legumes: snap beans, shell beans, peas, dry beans, and lentils

Moderate Purine Content: From 30 to 100 mg purine nitrogen in 100 gm or 90 to 300 mg/100 gm when calculated as uric acid

Meats except as noted	Fish, shellfish

High Purine Content: Over 100 mg purine nitrogen in 100 gm

Anchovies	Meat broth, gravies
Sardines	Meat extracts

Organ meats: Kidney, liver, sweetbreads, pancreas, brains

REFERENCES

Bayles, TB: Nutrition in diseases of the bones and joints. In Goodhart, RS; Shils, ME (Eds.): *Modern Nutrition in Health and Disease,* 5th ed. Philadelphia, Lea & Febiger, 1973, Chap 32.

Brazeau, P: Inhibitors of tubular transport of organic compounds. In Goodman, LS; Gilman, A (Eds.): *The Pharmacological Basis of Therapeutics,* 4th ed. New York, Macmillan, 1970.

Macklachlan, MJ; Rodnan, GP: Effects of food, fast, and alcohol on serum uric acid and acute attacks of gout. *Am J Med, 42*:38, 1967.

Mattice, MJ: *Bridges' Food and Beverage Analyses,* 3rd ed. Philadelphia, Lea & Febiger, 1950.

Mitchell, HS; Rynbergen, HJ; Anderson, L; Dibble, MV: *Cooper's Nutrition in Health and Disease,* 15th ed. Philadelphia, Lippincott, 1968, Chap 33.

Restegar, A; Thier, SO: The physiologic approach to hyperuricemia. *N Engl J Med, 286:*470, 1972.

Seegmiller, JE: Diseases of purine and pyrimidine metabolism. In Bondy, PK; Rosenberg, LE (Eds.): *Duncan's Diseases of Metabolism,* 6th ed. Philadelphia, Saunders, 1969, Chap 10.

MODIFICATIONS IN CONSTITUENTS:
B. FAT

" "THERE IS NO MORE *controversial field in all of clinical medicine than that which concerns the etiology, pathogenesis, prevention and treatment of atherosclerosis in general and coronary or ischemic heart disease in particular. It is generally agreed that the latter is a self-inflicted disease that is closely correlated with our American culture and way of life, but the relative importance of the various environmental factors continues to be vigorously debated. Epidemiological studies lead to widely diverse conclusions that confuse rather than clarify the problem.*

"Of all the environmental influences that have been identified, diet has probably received the greatest amount of attention, but here also, there is no agreement. Without any pretense at contributing any new information or opinions concerning these issues, it seems reasonable to state that diet is almost surely one factor out of many that influences the rate of development of the pathological changes of coronary artery disease. It may not be even the most important factor. It is also clear that individual patients differ metabolically in their sensitivity and responsiveness to alterations in therapeutic dietary manipulations, so that categorical statements concerning the importance of specific diets become virtually impossible.

"Recent new research information has refuted the previously accepted but tentative belief that the decline in blood cholesterol concentration induced by large dietary supplements of polyunsaturated fatty acids would be accompanied by a parallel improvement in morbidity and/or mortality in coronary heart disease. The fall in blood cholesterol level can easily and regularly be demonstrated but there is no comparable protective effect.

157

"Accordingly, it appears that these recommendations for increased amounts of polyunsaturates in the diet are no longer justified. These lipids, however, are still classified as 'essential' nutrients since they cannot be synthesized endogenously in adequate amounts but are metabolically indispensable. For this reason, the inclusion in these diets of some fats from non-animal sources (either margarine or vegetable oils) seems appropriate.

"With the intent to make this publication of maximum usefulness to the largest number of people, low fat, low saturated (animal) fat, and low cholesterol diets have been included with no bias as to their possible usefulness."

E. S. Gordon, M.D.

FAT CONTROLLED DIETS

The selection and quantity of fat in the diet is of concern in the following conditions.

1. To control calorie intake. The low calorie diets in the previous section are decreased in total fat content for weight control. A higher percentage of the total calories comes from protein sources. Carbohydrate and fat intake is controlled.

2. To meet the needs of the individual with a fat intolerance. This may be due to malabsorption or may be caused by gallbladder disease, pancreatitis or pancreatic insufficiency. Fat restriction is frequently recommended in treating acne.

3. To control cholesterol intake. This is achieved primarily by restriction of egg consumption, and the use of non-fat dairy foods (skim milk, low fat cottage cheese) and vegetable fat alternates (vegetable margarines instead of butter).

4. To decrease saturated fats in the diet in an effort to lower cholesterol in the blood. Most of these diets have controlled quantities of meat (and other sources of animal fats), and added quantities (if calories permit) of the vegetable oils which are relatively high in polyunsaturated fatty acids. The polyunsaturates have an hypocholesterolemic effect (Levy, et al, 1972).

Plans Included in This Section

The following dietary plans are included in this section:

1. A low fat diet. This restricts total fat to not more than 60 grams

per day. Either saturated or unsaturated fats may be used within the limits of the prescription. The ratio of polyunsaturates to saturates is not taken into consideration in this diet.

2. Five dietary regimens for use in the treatment of hyperlipoproteinemia (sometimes referred to as "Fredrickson diets" or "NIH diets"). Calories are decreased and cholesterol limited in four of these diets; carbohydrates are limited in three; the use of vegetable fats and oils rather than butter is recommended in four of the diets. These meal patterns have been adapted to midwestern food preferences for long term use. Cholesterol can be lowered and P/S ratio further increased by the elimination of egg, use of 1 teaspoon of safflower oil for each ounce of meat, and use of safflower oil soft margarine with a higher ratio of polyunsaturates than the average composition figure as shown from HG Bul No 72. Since processor's formulas change, recent composition data from the manufacturer is recommended.

Inspection of Table VI-21a, Comparison of Modified Fat Diets With Typical American Diet, will show how these diets have been modified. A list of the lipid values of some common foods is given in this section. Information on cholesterol, total saturated fat, oleic, and linoleic fatty acids is included.

LOW FAT DIET: NOT OVER 60 GRAMS FAT

Food consumption studies show that fat accounts for about 43% of the total calories consumed in the United States. Sixty grams of fat in a 2000 calorie diet provides 27% of the calories; in an 1800 calorie diet, 30% of the calories. The diet outline following provides 55 grams of fat or about 28% of an 1800 calorie diet. Diets with less than 25% of the calories from fat are not palatable. They are difficult to plan and are not well-received.

Indications for Use

The low fat diet may be of value for people with gallbladder disease for whom it is desirable to prevent stimulation of contractions of the gallbladder. It may also be used in pancreatitis, pancreatic insufficiency and some malabsorption syndromes.

Reduction of weight to normal is recognized as the single most important objective in reducing the risk factors of many diseases.

Reduction of fat consumption is one approach to a life-long pattern of controlled calorie intake.

All the low calorie diets in Section V are low fat diets. The quantities of lean meats, egg and free fats in the foods listed on these diets control the amount of fat. Milk of higher fat content (1 or 2% fat, or more) can be used if less fat restriction is required. Calories can be adjusted by adding fruits, vegetables and/or foods from the Bread-Cereal or Sweets group. The low calorie diets in Section V are lower in carbohydrate composition than the general consumption level in the United States.

People frequently cite intolerance to some foods that do not necessarily contain fat, but these intolerances vary from one individual to another. Therefore the foods termed "gas-forming," "strong-flavored," "dyspeptic," etc., that have traditionally been eliminated in fat restricted diets are not restricted in this diet. Individuals will omit those foods that cause distress.

It is important that a person understand that although symptoms

TABLE VI-11

LOW FAT DIET: 1800 CALORIES, NOT OVER 60 GRAMS FAT

Food Group	Amount	Protein gm	Fat gm	Corbohydrate gm	Calories
Milk, 2% butterfat	3 cups	30	15	45	435
Vegetables and fruit					
List A vegetables	Not limited		Negligible		
List B vegetables	2 exchanges	4	0	14	70
Fruit	4 exchanges	0	0	40	160
(Include a dark-green or deep yellow vegetable every other day, and a good source of vitamin C every day.)					
Bread-cereals					
Whole grain, enriched, or fortified	5 exchanges	10	0	75	350
Vegetables in bread-cereal group	2 exchanges	4	0	30	140
(Do not use ice cream.)					
Lean meat list (see Section I)	6 exchanges	48	18	0	360
Eggs (value 3/7)	3/week	3	2	0	34
(Count those used in cooking as well as those eaten as such.)					
Fats, oils*: animal or vegetable	4 teaspoons	0	20	0	180
Sweets: sugar, jelly, syrup, etc	4 teaspoons	0	0	16	67
Total		99	55	220	1,796
Percent of total calories		22%	28%	50%	

*If soft margarine (2 teaspoons) and corn oil (2 teaspoons) are used for the fats and oils, 10% of the calories will be from saturated fat; total cholesterol will be 324 mg. With such selection this pattern can be used for Type V hyperlipoproteinemia.

may appear following ingestion of a food, such symptoms may be independent of that particular food.

In cases of acute illness, the Soft Diet pattern may be followed in modifying the texture of the food offered.

Diet Pattern

Table VI-11 gives an example of a relatively low fat diet, less restricted in calories than the low calorie diets in Section V. Table VI-18, Diet Pattern According to Requirements for Type I Hyper-lipoproteinemia, is a diet severely restricted in fat, but with no attempt to change the P/S ratio. It is low in cholesterol.

POLYUNSATURATED FATS

Food fats contain saturated and unsaturated fatty acids; the un-saturates include mono-unsaturates (1 double bond) and polyun-saturates (fatty acids with more than 1 double bond). Linoleic acid constitutes the greatest proportion of polyunsaturates; there are few figures available for other polyunsaturates.

Animal foods containing fats (milk, meat, poultry, and their products) are higher in saturates than in polyunsaturates. To raise the ratio of polyunsaturates to saturates, animal products containing fat are restricted and vegetable oils containing a high ratio of poly-unsaturated fatty acids are included in the diet. Keys (1967) reported that oleic acid (1 double bond, mono-unsaturated) had little effect in raising or lowering serum cholesterol; and that the saturated fatty acids with 12 to 17 carbon atoms in the chain have a strong cholesterol-promoting action. Oleic acid constitutes about 40% of the total fat in foods consumed in the United States (Friend, 1970) but is not considered in calculating the P/S ratio.

For diets modified in fat and low in cholesterol, saturated free fats such as butter or solid vegetable shortenings should be avoided in food preparation; soft vegetable margarines and oils should be used instead. Vegetable margarines should be those with a P/S ratio of 1.5 or higher and with polyunsaturates constituting 30% or more of the total fat.

Emphasis on the reduction of saturated fats in the diet has stimulated production of soft margarines with a higher ratio of polyun-saturates. The percentage of total fat from polyunsaturated fatty acids in soft margarine is 37% in contrast to regular margarine

Diet in Health and Disease

which has 27% and whipped margarine 28% (calculated from H & G Bul No 72, 1970). Some "diet margarines" which are higher in polyunsaturates are being made. These soft ("tub") margarines are made from safflower oil or corn oil. Data on composition can be secured from the processor. Frequency of change makes listing here impossible.

Hydrogenation to make vegetable oils solid as for shortenings removes all or most of the unsaturated double bonds, thus making the product more saturated. For this reason the hydrogenated

TABLE VI-12

SATURATED, MONO- AND POLY-UNSATURATED FATS IN FOODS

From HG Bul #72: *Nutritive Value of Foods.* USDA, 1970.

See Table VI-13 for average values for meat and fish.

	Measure	Wt gm	Total Fat gm	Saturated gm	Fatty Acids Oleic gm	Linoleic gm
Milk, Cheese, Cream, and Similar Products						
Milk:						
Whole	1 cup	244	9	5	3	trace
Non-fat	1 cup	245	trace	—	—	—
2% fat + non-fat sol	1 cup	246	5	3	2	trace
Buttermilk	1 cup	245	trace	—	—	—
Cheese, natural:						
Cheddar	1 oz	28	9	5	3	trace
Cottage:						
Creamed	1 cup	245	10	6	3	trace
Uncreamed	1 cup	200	1	trace	trace	trace
Cream	2 tbsp	28	11	6	4	trace
Parmesan	1 tbsp	5	2	1	trace	trace
Swiss	1 oz	28	8	4	3	trace
Cheese, processed:						
American	1 oz	28	9	5	3	trace
Cheese food	1 tbsp	14	3	2	1	trace
Cheese spread	1 tbsp	14	3	2	1	trace
Cream:						
Half and Half (12% fat)	1 tbsp	15	2	1	1	trace
Light (18% fat)	1 tbsp	15	3	2	1	trace
Sour	1 tbsp	12	2	1	1	trace
Heavy (36% fat), whipped	1 tbsp	8	3	2	1	trace
Cream, imitation (made with veg fat)						
Powdered	1 tbsp	2	1	trace	trace	0
Liquid	1 tbsp	15	2	1	trace	0

TABLE VI-12 (Cont'd)

	Measure	Wt gm	Total Fat gm	Saturated gm	Fatty Acids Oleic gm	Linoleic gm
Whipped topping	1 tbsp	4	1	1	trace	0
Milk desserts						
Ice Cream:						
10% fat	1 cup	133	14	8	5	trace
16% fat	1 cup	148	24	13	8	1
Ice Milk:						
Hardened	1 cup	131	7	4	2	trace
Soft-serve	1 cup	175	9	5	3	trace
Yogurt						
Low fat	1 cup	245	4	2	1	trace
From whole milk	1 cup	245	8	5	3	trace
Eggs	1 egg	50	6	2	3	trace
Nuts						
Cashews	1 cup	140	64	11	45	4
Coconut, shredded	1 cup	130	46	39	3	trace
Peanuts	1 cup	144	72	16	31	21
Peanut butter	1 cup	16	8	2	4	2
Pecans	1 cup	108	77	5	48	15
Walnuts	1 cup	126	75	4	26	36
Grain products			Negligible in cereals and pastas. In baked products, depends on formula and fat used.			
Fats						
Butter	1 tsp	5	4	2	1	trace
Cooking fats:						
Lard	1 tbsp	13	13	5	6	1
Vegetable fat	1 tbsp	13	13	3	6	3
Margarine:						
Regular	1 tbsp	14	12	2	6	3
Soft	1 tbsp	14	11	2	4	4
Oils:						
Corn	1 tbsp	14	14	1	4	7
Cottonseed	1 tbsp	14	14	4	3	7
Olive	1 tbsp	14	14	2	11	10
Peanut	1 tbsp	14	14	3	7	4
Safflower	1 tbsp	14	14	1	2	10
Soybean	1 tbsp	14	14	2	3	7
French dressing	1 tbsp	16	6	1	1	3
Mayonnaise	1 tbsp	14	11	2	2	6
Salad dressing (Mayo type)	1 tbsp	15	6	1	1	3
Fruits						
Avocado, Calif	one	284	37	7	17	5
Other fruit				None		
Vegetables				None		

shortenings are excluded in diets where a high P/S ratio is desired. "Non-dairy" cream substitutes are generally high in saturated fatty acids (McIntire, 1971).

Home and Garden Bulletin No 72, *Nutritive Value of Foods* (1970) lists the saturated and unsaturated fatty acid composition of common portions of food. Handbook No 8, *Composition of Foods, Raw, Processed, Prepared* (Watt and Merrill, 1963) gives the composition in 100 gram portions. Table VI-13 provides a weighted average value for meats and fish which can be used if a definite ratio of polyunsaturated to saturated fats must be planned. Table VI-12 lists the saturated and unsaturated fat of a selected (from HG Bul No 72) group of foods.

In the low cholesterol, modified fat hospital diets for which nutrient estimates are made, corn oil was used for salad dressings. The averaged ratio of vitamin E (alpha-tocopherol) to polyunsaturates of the three diets was less than the 0.6 recommended by Harris and Embree (1963). Use of cottonseed oil instead of corn oil would have given a ratio above 0.6 milligram alpha-tocopherol per gram of linoleic acid as shown following.

Comparison of Ratios, Alpha-tocopherol to Linoleic Acid,
if Cottonseed Oil Were Used Instead of Corn Oil in Diet Plan

Low cholesterol, modified fat diets	*Alpha- tocopherol*	*Linoleic acid*	*Ratio*
	mg	gm	mg/gm
1200 calories: with corn oil	6.39	11.5	0.56
with cottonseed oil	8.46	11.5	0.74
1800 calories: with corn oil	8.40	15.8	0.53
with cottonseed oil	10.75	15.8	0.68

See Appendix I for references to the tocopherol composition of foods.

See Table VI-13 for fatty acids in lean meat, poultry, and fish.

CHOLESTEROL EXCHANGES AND CHOLESTEROL IN COMMON PORTIONS

Table VI-13 shows the rotation of meats, poultry and fish which average 25 mg cholesterol per ounce, ready-to-eat. Table VI-14 lists some foods in exchange groups according to similar cholesterol values. For flexibility in use, different kinds of milk and of fat are listed in the common units of use. Individuals tend to select a restricted number of products from each of these groups and to use these few products in a consistent pattern. Some of the items in the exchange groups (the uncreamed cottage cheese and shrimp, for example) are listed in portions greater than would normally be used. A fractional portion is expected to be used and the cholesterol value adjusted accordingly.

The derivation of the cholesterol value of the cheese is not shown. The value given for cured cheese represents an unweighted (for frequency of use) rounded average of the cured cheeses listed by Feeley, Criner, and Watt (1972), exclusive of the cottage cheese, ·rocessed cheese food and cheese spread listed separately. If a less varied selection is used frequently, the value of the cheese chosen might be appropriate. Cheddar, colby, and swiss average 27 to 28 mg cholesterol per ounce. Individual variation may be considerable.

Except for a few low-fat cheeses, most cured cheeses furnish between 90 to 100 mg cholesterol per 100 gms. Cheese *food* is slightly lower in cholesterol than either natural or processed cheese. Approximately 1-1/4 oz of processed american cheese *food* (20 mg cholesterol/oz) will furnish 25 mg cholesterol. Cheese *spread* yields only 18 mg cholesterol per oz, but in practical usage can be used in the same quantity as cheese food.

Cottage cheese is much lower in fat and cholesterol content than cured or processed cheeses. Creamed cottage cheese (4% fat) furnishes 48 mg cholesterol per cup; low fat cottage cheese (1% fat) yields 23 mg cholesterol per cup and uncreamed cottage cheese yields only 13 mg cholesterol per cup. Cream cheese is considerably higher in cholesterol content.

See Table A-1 Appendix I for some recent (1972) data on the cholesterol content of bacon, and of some sausage products as manufactured by the formula of one meat processor.

Some specially prepared low cholesterol filled-cheese products are on the market. These foods have the butterfat of natural cheese replaced with vegetable oil. One such product, Cheez-ola® (Trade name registered by Fisher Cheese Company, Wapakoneta, Ohio) is described as a filled, pasteurized process cheese containing 4.3 mg cholesterol per 100 grams with a P/S ratio of 4.5. The same company makes a 99 percent fat-free pasteurized cheese food-type

Diet in Health and Disease

TABLE VI-13—PROTEIN, FATS, AND CHOLESTEROL IN A SELECTED GROUP
OF LEAN MEATS, POULTRY, AND FISH

Meats, poultry, fish, cooked. Separable lean parts only.	Protein[1] gm	Total gm	Fats[1] Saturated gm	Oleic gm	Linoleic gm	Cholesterol[2] mg
Beef: 1 ounce						
Pot roast, braised	8.4	2.0	0.8	2.0	Trace	25
Rib, roasted	7.8	3.9	1.7	2.0	"	25
Round, roasted	8.7	1.1	0.4	0.4	"	25
Steak, round, broiled	8.8	1.7	0.8	0.4	"	25
Steak, sirloin, broiled	9.0	2.0	1.0	1.0	"	25
Ground (lean hamburger)	7.7	3.3	1.7	1.3	"	25
Dried or chipped beef	9.5	2.0	1.0	1.0	"	26[3]
Lamb: 1 ounce						
Leg, roasted	8.0	2.0	1.2	0.8	"	28
Shoulder, roasted	**7.4**	**2.6**	1.3	0.9	"	28
Pork, lean cuts: 1 ounce						
Pork, fresh, roasted	8.3	4.2	1.3	1.7	0.4	25
Pork, fresh, simmered	8.2	2.7	0.9	1.4	0.5	25
Pork, fresh chop, lean part	8.8	4.1	1.2	1.8	0.6	25
Cured ham, boiled	5.5	5.0	2.0	2.0	0.5	25
Veal, medium fat: 1 ounce						
Cutlet, no bone	7.7	3.0	1.7	1.3	Trace	28
Round, roasted	7.7	4.7	2.3	2.0	"	28
Poultry: 1 ounce						
Chicken, all classes and cuts, flesh and skin	6.7	1.0	0.3	0.3	0.3	24
Turkey, light meat	9.0	1.7	0 6	0.3 (raw)	0.3 (raw)	22
Fish[4]: 1-1/2 ounces cooked weight						
Haddock, fried	8.5	2.6	0.5	1.5	Trace	25[5]
Salmon, red, canned solids and liquid	8.5	5.9	1.7	1.7	"	15
Tuna, canned in oil, drained solids	12.0	3.5	1.1	1.7	0.5	27
Totals, 20 items	166.2	59.0	23.5	26.5	3.1	501
Averages	8.3	3.0	1.2	1.3	0.2	25
Rounded to	8.0	3.0	1.2	1.3	0.2	25

[1]Protein and fat values from Home and Garden Bulletin #72 (1970) and are for the cooked product.

[2]Cholesterol values (except dried beef) from Feeley, RM; Criner, PE; Watt, BK: Cholesterol content of food. *J Am Diet Assoc, 61*:134, 1972. Use of copyright data courtesy of American Dietetic Association and the authors. All values for cooked product unless otherwise noted

[3]From *Mayo Clinic Dietetic Manual* (1971).

[4]Items included in average above are representative. Fish items between 35 and 65 mg cholesterol per 100 gms as listed by Feeley, Criner and Watt average 52 mg cholesterol per 100 gm (22 mg per 1-1/2 oz). The average value includes drained canned clams, fresh raw cod, raw flounder, raw haddock, fresh raw oysters drained, broiled salmon steak, canned red salmon solids and liquids, steamed scallops, raw flesh of trout and drained solids of tuna canned in oil.

[5]Cholesterol value is for fresh raw haddock flesh.

Table VI-14 Cholesterol Exchanges and Cholesterol in Common Portions of Food. Data from Freeley, RM; Criner, PE; Watt, BK: Cholesterol content of food, *J Am Diet Assoc, 61*:134, 1972. Courtesy of the authors and the American Dietetic Association.

Meats, Poultry, and Fish. One exchange in quantity listed furnishes 25 mg cholesterol. All meats cooked. Organ meats not included in this exchange. See Table VI-13 for frequency weighting of cuts used in establishing average cholesterol values.

	Quantity to furnish 25 mg cholesterol
Meats	1 ounce
Beef, any cut	
Lamb, any cut	
Pork, any cut	
Veal, any cut	
Chicken, all classes, flesh and skin	
Turkey, light meat	
Fish (including some shellfish)—low cholesterol	1-1/2 ounce
Any not listed below or in cholesterol exchanges	
for egg yolk. See Table VI-13, footnote 4 for	
items included in establishing average cholesterol value.	
Fish—higher cholesterol	1 ounce
(85 to 105 mg cholesterol per 100 gm)	
Includes crabmeat (steamed fresh, or canned drained),	
herring (raw flesh or plain canned solids and liquids),	
lobster (cooked meat),	
and mackerel (raw or canned solids and liquids).	

Cheeses. One exchange (quantity in last column) provides 25 mg cholesterol.

	Quantity to furnish 25 mg cholesterol
Cured or processed, any kind	1 ounce
Cheese food, pasteurized processed american	1-1/4 ounce
Cheese spread, pasteurized processed american	1-1/3 ounce
Cottage cheese:	

	Household Measure	Weight gm	Cholesterol In Household Measure	In 100 gm	
1% fat	1 cup	267	23	9	1 cup
4 % fat	1 cup	245	48	19	1/2 cup
Uncreamed	1 cup	200	13	7	2 cups
Cream cheese	1 tbsp	14	16	111	1-1/2 tbsp

Egg, Organ Meats and High Cholesterol Fish. One exchange = 250 mg cholesterol. Exchange value based on cholesterol content of yolk from one large egg (egg without shell 50 gm; yolk 17 gm, cholesterol 252 mg).

Organ Meats, cooked	Cholesterol/100 gm mg	Quantity to furnish 250 mg cholesterol
Gizzard, chicken	195	4-1/2 ounce
Heart: beef	274	3-1/4 ounce
chicken	231	4 ounces
Kidney: beef, calf, hog,		
or lamb	804	1 ounce

Table VI-14 (Continued)

Liver: beef, calf, hog,		
or lamb	438	2 ounces
chicken	746	1-1/4 ounce
Sweetbreads	466	2 ounces
Brains	<2000	not used due to high content

Fish—(over 125 mg cholesterol per 100 gm)

Caviar (1 tbsp = 16 gm)	300	5-1/4 tbsp
Shrimp, raw flesh or canned drained		
solids	150	6 ounces

Milk, Cream, and Ice Cream (See Fats for sour and whipping cream)

This is not an exchange list.

	Household Measure	Wt gm	Cholesterol (mg) in	
			Household Measure	100 gm
Buttermilk, non-fat	1 cup	245	5	2
Chocolate milk drink	1 cup	250	20	8
Cream				
Half and half (12% fat)	1 tbsp	15	6	43
	1 cup	242	105	
light (18% fat)	1 tbsp	15	10	66
	1 cup	240	158	
Ice cream				
10% fat	1 cup	133	53	40
16% fat (approx)	1 cup	148	85	57
Frozen custard	1 cup	133	97	73
Ice milk				
Hardened	1 cup	131	26	20
Soft serve	1 cup	175	36	20
Milk				
whole—3.5% fat	1 cup	244	34	14
1% fat + 1-2% non fat solids	1 cup	246	14	6
2% fat + 1-2% non-fat solids	1 cup	246	22	9
Non-fat (skim)	1 cup	245	5	2
Canned evaporated, undil	1 cup	252	79	31
Canned, condensed, undil	1 cup	306	105	34
Dry, reconstituted	1 cup		5	2
Yogurt				
Plain or vanilla, non-fat	8 oz carton	227	17	8
Fruit flavored	8 oz carton	227	15	7

Fats. Cholesterol value of common portions. | Not an exchange list. |

	Household Measure	Wt gm	Cholesterol (mg) in	
Table fats				
Butter, regular	1 pat (1 tsp)	5	12	250
	1 tbsp	14	35	250
Butter, whipped	1 tbsp	9	22	250
Cream, sour 18% fat	1 tbsp	12	8	66
	1 cup	230	152	66
Whipped topping, pressurized	1 cup	60	51	85

Table VI-14 (Continued)

	Household Measure	Wt gm	Cholesterol (mg) in Household Measure	100 gm
Whipping cream (37% fat)				
Unwhipped	1 tbsp	15	20	133
	1 cup	238	316	133
Whipped	about doubles in bulk			
Margarine				
All vegetable				0
Mixed fat: 2/3 animal,				
1/3 vegetable	1 tbsp	14	7	50
Mayonnaise, commercial	1 tsp	5	3	23
	1 tbsp	14	10	70
Salad dressing,				
mayonnaise type	1 tsp	5	3	17
	1 tbsp	15	8	50
Oil, vegetable, any kind				0
Other fats				
Chicken fat (raw)				65
Lard	1 cup	205	195	95
Shortening, all vegetable				0

Foods that have negligible or no cholesterol content:

These foods can be used freely limited only by the calorie, P/S ratio, and/or protein prescription.

Olive oil, coconut, avocados and solid cooking fats contain a higher ratio of saturated fatty acids, but, like all vegetable products, are cholesterol free.

Dry cottage cheese (non-fat)—12 mg cholesterol per 1/2 cup.

Egg white—no cholesterol.

Non-fat buttermilk—5 mg cholesterol per cup.

Skim milk—5 mg cholesterol per cup.

All fruits and vegetables and all-vegetable products—no cholesterol.

Peanut butter (about 1/4 saturated fat, 1/2 oleic acid and 1/4 linoleic acid) —no cholesterol.

Vegetable oils and products made from vegetable oils with no animal fats.

product for low fat, low cholesterol diets. It contains only 5 mg cholesterol per 100 grams. Other similar products are advertised.

Low cholesterol egg products are available. Some of these dilute the cholesterol content of the whole egg by adding additional egg white. Others remove the fat from the egg yolk and add flavoring ingredients and emulsifiers.

A very acceptable scrambled egg or egg salad mixture of lower cholesterol content can be made by using 1/3 to 1/2 egg yolk only per total white of each egg. By this method in group feeding it is important that the serving portion be controlled. Whole eggs are approximately 30 percent yolk, 59 percent white and 11 percent shell. Cost comparisons with the commercial low cholesterol egg alternates will reveal whether discarding some of the yolks is an

TABLE VI-15

AVERAGE VALUES OF FOOD GROUPS USED IN PLANNING LOW CHOLESTEROL, MODIFIED FAT DIETS

Refer to food exchange lists for size of servings.

Food group	Amount	Protein gm	Fats — Total gm	Fats — Saturated gm	Linoleic Acid gm	Cholesterol mg	Carbohydrate gm	Calories
Milk, skim	8 ounce cup	8	—	—	—	5	12	80
Vegetables								
List 2A	Not limited						Negligible	
List 2B	1 exchange	2	0	0	0	0	7	35
Fruit	1 exchange	0	0	0	0	0	10	40
Bread-cereals	1 exchange	2	0	0	0	0	15	70
Lean meat, fish (from Table VI-13)	1 ounce	8	3	1.2	0.2	25	0	60
Egg	One	6	6	2.0	Trace	252	0	75
Peanut butter	1 tablespoon	4	8	2.0	2.0	0	3	95
Fats, vegetable								
Margarine, soft	1 teaspoon	0	4	0.7	1.3	0	0	36
Oil, corn	1 teaspoon	0	5	0.3	2.3	0	0	45
Sweets	1 tablespoon	0	0	0	0	0	12	50

There need be no calculation other than the correct number of exchanges when meats or fish are chosen from Table VI-13. Other foods may be used if calculated within the limits of the P/S ratio, cholesterol, and calorie level prescribed. Sweets are calculated at 50 calories for a tablespoon and include honey, jelly, jam, preserves, molasses, table syrups, and any kind of sugar. Distribute their use among the day's meals. Use mainly as a flavoring ingredient in combined foods such as custards, puddings, and baked goods.

economic solution to achieving a lower cholesterol intake. Desired frequency of use and flavor acceptability undoubtedly will influence the selection which will limit cholesterol intake to the desired range.

There is much individual variation in the cholesterol content of eggs. Selection of a smaller egg, "medium" (21 to 24 oz per doz) or "small" (18 to 21 oz per doz) size, does not always give a decrease in cholesterol content porportional to the lesser weight.

The cholesterol of eggs is found in the yolk. The white is cholesterol free. In most baked goods two egg whites can generally be substituted for one whole egg.

Official analytical methods as well as market products are changing, so comparison of older food composition data with the more recent is not always valid. Most older data represents total sterols, whereas some recent data is for cholesterol only.

Advertisements in the *Journal of the American Dietetic Association* and the *Journal of the American Medical Association,* and a search under "cholesterol" of the index issues of these journals will note current technological developments in the production of low cholesterol foods.

LOW CHOLESTEROL, MODIFIED FAT DIETS

These diets represent one approach to controlling serum lipids, atherosclerosis, and associated heart disease. Short term use of these diets is rarely effective in altering blood chemistry. All of the diets, except Type I of the Diets for the Five Types of Hyperlipoproteinemia (Table VI-18) have an increased ratio of polyunsaturated fats and are restricted in cholesterol. Polyunsaturates aid in lowering blood cholesterol.

Cholesterol is found in animal products. Eggs, dairy fats, organ meats, caviar, and shrimp are particularly rich sources of cholesterol. Some of the cholesterol in meats is bound to the protein, so it is impossible to achieve cholesterol-free meats. Skim milk contains some cholesterol. See Table VI-13 for cholesterol in common foods. The fat composition of commercial baked foods is so variable that no attempt was made to include them in this listing, or in the listing of saturated and polyunsaturated fats.

The term "modified fat diet" generally refers to modifying the ordinary dietary selection of fats to achieve a higher ratio of polyunsaturated fats in the diet.

To increase the ratio of polyunsaturated to saturated fats in the diet (P/S ratio), changes in the typical American eating pattern are necessary. The average P/S ratio in United States is 0.41 (Friend, 1970) according to civilian consumption statistics. The following changes are generally made to achieve a higher ratio of polyunsaturated fats:

1. Use non-fat milk only.
2. Use only lean meats trimmed of visible fats. Even lean meat is relatively high in saturated fats and intake must be controlled if a high P/S ratio is to be achieved at a modest calorie level. Frequent use of meat alternates such as cheese and eggs which are high in saturated fats is not recommended if a high P/S ratio is desired. Nuts vary in the proportion of unsaturated fats. Walnuts are high in polyunsaturated fats and are recommended if a high P/S ratio is desired (and calories allow). Coconut and coconut oil are high in saturates and would be avoided. Eggs are limited to 3 per week, or less. In addition to being rich in saturated fat, the yolk is very high in cholesterol.
3. Plain fats (table and cooking fats) should be oils and the softer all-vegetable fats. Hydrogenation to make fats more solid reduces the percent of unsaturated fatty acids present. Vegetable fats vary in their quantity and ratio of polyunsaturates to saturates. Safflower oil and corn oil, and the soft margarines made from these oils, are relatively high in polyunsaturates and are very useful if a high P/S ratio must be achieved. The margarines have a lower P/S ratio than the oils. If no other sources of fat are included in the diet (such as eggs, cream, or cream soups or rich desserts), use of 1 teaspoon of corn oil (45 calories) per ounce of cooked lean meat (60 calories) will result in approximately a 1.7 ratio; if safflower oil is used instead of corn oil this ratio will be approximately 2.4. Where calories are severely restricted, use of 1/2 teaspoon of safflower oil (23 calories) per ounce of lean cooked meat will give a P/S ratio of 1.4 if no sources of saturated fat other than the lean meat and the oil are included in the diet. Eggs are high in saturated fat and will affect the P/S ratio as well as the cholesterol content of the diet. Where a high protein, or a very low calorie diet acceptable to patients is the first goal, a high P/S ratio is not

possible. Vegetable oils must be used to increase the ratio of unsaturates and they increase calories. With even a P/S ratio of 1, use of cheese, eggs, cream soups and commercial baked goods is very limited. Most margarines do not have as high a P/S ratio as liquid corn oil.

4. Fruits and vegetables (exclusive of avocados, coconuts, and olives) are fat free and can be used freely without altering the P/S ratio. Most cereal products of the bread-cereal group are practically fat-free and can be used freely unless carbohydrates must be controlled. However, commercially baked pastries, desserts, and combined entrees of unknown formula are best avoided. They will probably contain considerable animal fats or hydrogenated fats. Desserts prepared with vegetable oil and foods fried in vegetable oil can be used if carbohydrates and calories are not limited.

5. A considerable proportion of the fatty acids of chocolate, coconut and olive oil are saturated, so these products will change the P/S ratio. They are cholesterol free. Many condensed soups, which may be used frequently, are made with milk solids and can be expected to carry some cholesterol as well as saturated fats. Where a high P/S ratio is desired, these foods are not used except as calculated in the diet.

Quantitative limitation of cholesterol and saturated fatty acids requires calculation of the diet in order to fit the customs, family pattern of meals, likes and dislikes of foods, and the economic level of the person for whom it is prescribed. It should be noted that restrictions must remain fairly rigid in order to accomplish the purpose of the dietary changes.

Medium chain triglycerides may be used in food preparation for Type I hyperlipoproteinemia (very low fat) diet. They are an edible oil product prepared chemically from the fatty acids of 6 to 12 carbons. Differences in the way the body transports and utilizes them in contrast to ordinary fats has led to their use in some conditions of fat intolerance. They are "fatless fats." They provide carbon and hydrogen for energy at the rate of 8 calories per gram and are oxidized to acetate (Senior, 1968, page 249). Medium chain triglyceride oil is sold by pharmacies. For information about its use see Schizas, et al (1967) and the list of commercial sources of special foods in Appendix IV.

TABLE VI-16

CALCULATED NUTRIENT ESTIMATES OF DIETS MODIFIED IN FAT AS SERVED IN A HOSPITAL

Nutrients	*Unit*	*Recommended Dietary Allowances*		*Low Fat Diet*	*Hospital Diets*	
		Man 23-50 Years Old	*Woman 23-50 Years Old*		*Modified Fat Diet Low Cholesterol 1,200 Calories*	*Modified Fat Diet Low Cholesterol 1,800 Calories*
Food energy	Calorie	2,700	2,000	1,670	1,230	1,860
Protein	gm	56	46	95	85	100
Fat	gm	—	—	55	45	65
Carbohydrate	gm	—	—	215	125	220
Calcium	gm	0.8	0.8	1.3	0.8	0.9
Phosphorus	gm	0.8	0.8	1.5	1.3	1.5
Iron	mg	10.0	18.0	15.0	11.0	15.0
Magnesium	mg	350	300	326	226	281
Sodium	mg	—	—	2,140	2,747	3,315
Sodium mEq				93	119	144
Potassium	mg	—	—	3,397	3,077	3,720
Potassium mEq				87	79	95
Vitamin A	IU	5,000	4,000	9,390	6,076	6,701
Vitamin E	IU	15 IU	12 IU	5.4 mg	6.4 mg	8.4
Ascorbic acid	mg	45.0	45.0	93.0	95.0	121.0
Folacin	mg	0.4	0.4	—	—	—
Niacin equivalent	mg	18.0	13.0	32.0	29.0	35.0
Riboflavin	mg	1.6	1.2	2.9	1.8	2.2
Thiamin	mg	1.4	1.0	1.4	1.4	1.7
Vitamin B_6	mg	2.0	2.0	3.0	1.9	2.3
Vitamin B_{12}	mcg	3.0	3.0	5.8	4.2	4.8

Holt (DM: *Disease-a-Month*, June 1971) and Gracey, et al (*Arch Dis Child, 45*:445, 1970) described disorders in fat absorption in children and adults which respond to treatment with medium chain triglycerides. Bowman (1973) described factors influencing the quality and acceptability of products baked with medium chain triglycerides. Howard and Morse (1973) presented formulas for muffins and pastry.

DIETARY MANAGEMENT IN HYPERLIPOPROTEINEMIA

Fredrickson and co-workers of the National Institutes of Health separated the hyperlipoproteinemias into five (now six, with the separation of type II into two parts) types as follows on the basis of abnormalities in the lipoprotein components.

Classification of Hyperlipoproteinemias, Serum Abnormalities, and Response to Diet. Adapted from Levy and Fredrickson (1968) and Levy, et al (1972).

Type	Lipoprotein	Triglycerides	Cholesterol	Response to Alterations In Carbohydrate	In Fat
I	Severe Chylomicronemia	Elevated	Normal or elevated	None	Yes
IIa	LDL increased normal VLDL	Normal	Elevated	None	Slight
IIb	LDL increased + excess VLDLP	Elevated		Glucose intolerance	
III	VLDL/LDL of abnormal composition	Elevated	Elevated	Glucose intolerance	Yes
IV	VLDL increased normal or decreased LDL	Elevated	Normal or elevated	Glucose intolerance	None
V	Chylomicrons present. VLDL increased	Elevated	Elevated or normal	Most patients have glucose intolerance	Yes

LDL = low density (beta) lipoproteins
VLDL = very low density (pre-beta) lipoproteins

Lipoproteins are classified on the basis of their separation either by electrophoresis or ultracentrifugation. Levy, et al (1972) described the composition of the various fractions.

Composition of Lipoprotein Families
Compiled from data by Levy, R. L., et al: *Ann Intern Med, 77*:267-294, 1972.

Lipoprotein Family	Protein	Composition Phospholipid	Triglyceride	Cholesterol
Chylomicrons	1-2%	3-6%	80-90%	2-7%
Very low density lipoproteins (VLDL; pre-beta LP)	5-10%	15-20%	55-60%	10-15%
Low density lipoproteins (LDL; beta LP)	25%	22%	10%	45%
High density lipoproteins (LDL; alpha LP)	45-50%	30%	Little	20%

Levy, et al (1972) explained the origin and diagnostic value of the 4 families of lipoproteins as follows:

Chylomicrons are synthesized in the intestines. They transport the triglycerides from food sources to the plasma and ultimately to the tissues. Normally they clear from the plasma in 8 to 10 hours.

The very low density lipoproteins (VLDL) transport the triglycerides (TG) which are synthesized in the liver from fatty acids and carbohydrate, or are derived from body stores. The intestines also synthesize some VLDL. In the absence of chylomicrons, an increase in VLDL is correlated with an increase in TG as shown in the chart. Both chylomicrons and VLDL are rich sources of TG and an increase in either or both may produce hypertriglyceridemia. Excess calories, a high carbohydrate diet, and alcohol exacerbate hyperglyceridemia.

Low density lipoproteins (LDL) are formed from the intravascular breakdown of VLDL. They normally carry the major portion of cholesterol in fasting plasma.

High density lipoproteins are normally present in fasting plasma. Their function is unclear.

A complete fast for 12 to 14 hours is essential to secure a meaningful lipoprotein analysis. All beverages (even black coffee) and cigarettes are to be avoided during this period. Water is allowed.

Different values have been quoted for safe (vs "normal") levels of triglyceride and cholesterol. There is some variation according to the population group and age. The upper limit for triglyceride is generally recognized as 150 mg/100 ml, with some increase with age (never over 160 mg/100 ml, or at the most 170 mg/100 ml in the elderly). A cholesterol value over 260 mg/100 ml plasma is generally cause for concern. Blood cholesterol values increase with age.

Dietary management is based on correcting lipoprotein abnormalities. If there is a severe chylomicronemia (excess chylomicrons in the blood), dietary fats are decreased. An increase in endogenous triglycerides (elevated VLDL after a 14 hour fast) is treated by weight reduction and a diet restricted in carbohydrates (including alcohol). If LDLP which are high in cholesterol are elevated, a diet low in cholesterol and saturated fats, with increased poly-

Adapted from *The Dietary Management of Hyperlipoproteinemia: A Handbook for Physicians* (Fredrickson, DS, et al. Revised 1971) and Levy, RI, et al: Dietary and drug treatment of primary hyperlipoproteinemia. *Am Intern Med,* 77:267, 1972.

Type	Protein foods	Fats	Carbohydrate	Cholesterol	Calories
I See Table VI-18	Meats limited due to fat limitation.	Total fat not more than 25 to 35 grams from all food. P/S ratio not considered.	Not restricted in kind or amount. Alcohol not recommended.	Not restricted.	Adjusted to requirement for ideal weight.
IIa See Table VI-19	Limited in kind and amount by restriction in cholesterol and saturated fat only.	Saturated fat intake restricted, polyunsaturated fat increased to a P/S ratio from 1.8 to 2.8 if calories allow.	Not restricted, 40-65% of total calories. Limited use of alcohol allowed.	Restricted: 300 mg or less per day.	Calories usually not restricted.
IIb See Table VI-19	Same	Same	Same, except weight reduction may require carbohydrate control to less than 40 percent of total calories.		Weight reduction often indicated.
III See Table VI-19	18 to 21% of total calories with cholesterol limitation.	40 to 45% of total calories. Restrict saturated fats.	Controlled: 36 to 41% of total calories. No concentrated sweets. Alcohol restricted.	Restricted to 300 mg or less per day.	To achieve and maintain ideal weight.
IV See Table VI-19	Limited only by cholesterol and calorie allowance.	P/S ratio not emphasized but cholesterol control will require animal fat restriction.	Controlled: 40-45% of total calories. Concentrated sweets avoided. Alcohol restricted.	300 to 500 mg per day.	To achieve and maintain ideal weight.
V See Table VI-20	High protein: 21 to 24% of total calories. Limited in kind by cholesterol allowance.	Limited to 25 to 30% of total calories; less when symptoms are acute. Select polyunsaturated fats when possible.	Controlled: about 50% of total calories. Avoid concentrated sweets and alcohol.	300 to 500 mg per day.	To achieve and maintain ideal weight.

The 85 page booklet, *Dietary Management of Hyperlipoproteinemia: A Handbook for Physicians,* is available (1973) upon request to the Office of Heart Information, National Heart Lung Institute, Building 31, Room 4A10, National Institutes of Health, Bethesda, Maryland, 20014. Separate booklets on each of the five types of hyperlipoproteinemias are available upon request for patient instruction.

TABLE VI-18

DIET PATTERN ACCORDING TO REQUIREMENTS FOR TYPE I HYPERLIPOPROTEINEMIA

Adapted from Fredrickson, DS, et al: *Dietary Management of Hyperlipoproteinemia: Handbook for Physicians*, revised. Bethesda, Maryland, Natl Heart and Lung Institute, NIH, 1971.

	Amount	Protein gm	Fat Total gm	Fat Saturated gm	Fat Unsaturated gm	Carbohydrate gm	Calories
Milk, skim	3 cups	24	—			36	240
Vegetables							
List 2A, Page 16	Not limited		Negligible				
List 2B, Page 17	2 exchanges	4	0			14	70
Fruit	4 exchanges	0	0			40	160
Bread-cereal group							
Breads or cereals	5 exchanges	10	0			75	350
Starchy vegetables	3 exchanges	6	0			45	210
Lean meat, poultry, or fish	6 exchanges (6 oz)	48	18	7.2	1.2	0	360
Egg (3/7) value	3 per week	3	2	1.0	tr	0	34
Fats, oils (animal or vegetable) calculated as							
Margarine	1 teaspoon	0	4	0.7	1.3	0	45
Oil, corn	1 teaspoon	0	5	0.3	2.3	0	45
Sweets							
Sugar, jelly, syrups, etc.	3 tablespoons					36	150
(Allow 1 teaspoon for each exchange of sweetened fruit)							
Total		95	29	(9.2)	(4.8)	246	1664
Percent of total calories		23%	16%	(5%)	(2.6%)	61%	

TABLE VI-19

DIET PATTERN ACCORDING TO REQUIREMENTS FOR TYPE II b HYPERLIPOPROTEINEMIA*—1400 CALORIES

Adapted from Fredrickson, DS, et al: *Dietary Management of Hyperlipoproteinemia: Handbook for Physicians*, revised, Bethesda, Maryland. Natl Heart and Lung Institute, NIH, 1971.

Food group	Amount	Protein gm	Total Fat gm	Saturated Fat gm	Linoleic Acid gm	Carbohydrate gm	Cholesterol mg	Calories
Milk, skim	2 cups	16	trace	—	—	24	10	160
Meat, lean, cooked	5 exchanges	40	15	6.0	1.0	—	125	300
Bread-cereal group	4 exchanges	8	—	—	—	60	0	280
A vegetables	As desired	—	0	0	0	—	0	—
B vegetables	2 exchanges	4	0	0	0	14	0	70
Fruit	3 exchanges	—	0	0	0	30	0	120
Fats (From Handbook 8, 1963. Pages 133 and 135)								
Vegetable margarines, soft	5 teaspoons (25 gm)	0	20	3.5	6.5	0	0	180
Vegetable oil (safflower)	5 teaspoons (25 gm)	0	25	1.5	16.5	0	0	225
Sweets	1 tablespoon (18 gm)	0	0	0	0	12	0	50
Totals		68	60	(11.0)	(24.0)	140	135	1385
Percent of total calories		20%	40%	(7%)	(15.6%)	40%		

P/S Ratio: 2.2 when safflower oil is used, 1.7 when corn oil is used.
*This same pattern can be followed for Type IIa, III and IV.

TABLE VI-20

DIET PATTERN ACCORDING TO REQUIREMENTS FOR TYPE V HYPERLIPOPROTEINEMIA — APPROX 1800 CALORIES

Adapted from Fredrickson, DS, et al: *Dietary Management of Hyperlipoproteinemia: Handbook for Physicians*, revised. Bethesda, Maryland, Natl Heart and Lung Institute, NIH, 1971.

Food group	Amount	Protein gm	Total Fat gm	Saturated Fat gm	Linoleic Acid gm	Carbohydrate gm	Cholesterol mg	Calories
Milk, skim	2 cups	16	—			24	10	160
Vegetables								
List 2A, page 16	No limit				Negligible			
List 2B, page 17	2 exchanges	4	0	0	0	14	0	70
Fruit	5 "	0	0	0	0	50	0	200
Bread-cereal group								
Grain foods	6 "	12	—	—	—	90	0	420
Vegetables, starchy	3 "	6	0	0	0	45	0	210
Cholesterol exchanges								
Lean meat, poultry, fish	8 "	64	24	9.6	1.6	0	200	480
Eggs (value 3/7)	3 per week	3	2	2.0	trace	0	108	34
Fats, vegetable								
Margarine, soft	3 teaspoons	0	12	2.1	3.9	0	0	108
Oil, corn	3 "	0	15	0.9	6.9	0	0	135
Totals		105	53	(14.6)	(12.4)	223	318	1817
Percent of total calories		24%	27%	(7.4%)	(6.2%)	49%		

P/S ratio: 0.8 when using products listed in Table VII-5; 1.0 when safflower oil is used, no change in margarines.
Cholesterol is within diet prescription of 300 to 500 mg daily.
1 tablespoon sugar or other sweet can be used in place of one exchange from the bread-cereal group.

TABLE VI-21a

COMPARISON OF MODIFIED FAT DIETS WITH TYPICAL AMERICAN DIET

The percentage distribution of calories from protein, fat, and carbohydrate in the civilian usage of foods (Friend, 1970). P/S ratio and cholesterol compared with similar figures for diets in which the fat content is controlled.

Table	Protein	Percent of Total Calories From: Fat Total	Saturated*	Carbohydrate	PS/Ratio*	Cholesterol* mg
Civilian use in the United States, 1969	12%	42%	14%	46%	0.4	500 to 1000
Hospital general diet described in Section II	15%	38%		47%	Variable	370 to 450
Conventional decreased calorie diets:						
V-3 1029 calories (prescribed 1000 calories)	27%	28%	3.3%	45%	0.9	245*
V-4 1204 calories (prescribed 1200 calories)	27%	30%	7.6%	43%	0.9	270*
V-5 1509 calories (prescribed 1500 calories)	23%	30%	6.0%	47%	0.9	280 to 300*
Multi-meal decreased calorie diets: These are high protein, moderate fat, reduced carbohydrate.						
V-7A 1195 calories (Plan A, 1200 calories)	36%	42%	12%	22%	0.6	370 to 510**
V-7B 1075 calories (Plan B, 1000 calories)	39%	43%	13%	18%	0.4	350 to 500**
V-7C 1067 calories (Plan C, 1000 calories)	34%	39%	11%	27%	0.5	320 to 450**
Low fat diet, not over 60 grams fat: (No modification of P/S ratio.)						
VII-1 1796 calories (1800 calorie diet)	22%	28%	10%	50%	0.8	324
Diets for Hyperlipoproteinemia:						
VII-7 Type I Very low fat, high carbohydrate	23%	16%	5%	61%	0.5 to 0.6†	275
VII-8 Type II Controlled fat, reduced carbohydrate, high P/S ratio	20%	40%	7%	40%	1.7 to 2.2†	135
VII-9 Type V Low fat, moderately high carbohydrate	24%	27%	7%	49%	0.8 to 1.0†	320

*Approximate values when all selections from the Fats and Oils group are vegetable oils or margarine as listed in Table VII-5.

**Three eggs per week in addition to the meat would yield the lower cholesterol value; one egg daily in addition to the meat would result in the higher cholesterol content.

†Higher ratio when safflower oil is used for 1/2 of the fat exchanges or when special high ratio "diet margarine" is used.

TABLE VI-21b

FATTY ACIDS AVAILABLE PER CAPITA PER DAY AND PERCENT OF TOTAL NUTRIENT FAT ACCOUNTED FOR BY FATTY ACIDS, SELECTED PERIODS

Year	Total Saturated gms	Fatty Acids Unsaturated[1] Oleic Acid gms	Linoleic Acid gms	Total Nutrient Fat gms	Share of Total Fat From Fatty Acids Total Saturated %	Oleic Acid %	Linoleic Acid %
1909-1913	50.3	51.5	10.7	125.2	40.2	41.1	8.5
1925-1929	53.3	55.2	12.5	134.6	39.6	41.0	9.3
1935-1939	52.9	54.5	12.7	133.0	39.8	41.0	9.5
1947-1949	54.4	58.0	14.8	141.1	38.6	41.1	10.5
1957-1959	54.7	58.2	16.6	143.2	38.2	40.6	11.6
1965	53.9	58.8	19.1	144.8	37.2	40.6	13.2
1970[2]	55.5	62.8	22.8	155.2	35.8	40.5	14.7

[1]Major unsaturated fatty acids. Oleic is mono-unsaturated and linoleic is poly-unsaturated.
[2]Preliminary.
Friend, B: Nutritional review. *National Food Situation* NFS-134, Econ Res Serv, USDA, Washington, DC, US Govt Printing Office, 1970.

unsaturated fats, is prescribed. The polyunsaturates have a cholesterol clearing effect.

Beaumont, JL, et al (*Bul WHO, 43*:891, 1970) described criteria for the differential diagnosis of the different types of hyperlipoproteinemias.

NATIONWIDE CHANGES IN CONSUMPTION OF FAT AND CARBOHYDRATE

Trends in the civilian use of fats in the United States are shown by statistics of foods available for consumption compiled by the US Department of Agriculture (Friend, 1970 and 1971). These studies show that the per capita per day consumption of fat from all food sources has increased from 125.2 grams in the 1909-13 base period to 155.2 grams in 1970 (Table VI-21b).

The ratio of polyunsaturated fatty acids to saturated fatty acids (PUFA/S or P/S) also changed during this period. In the 1909-13 period the ratio was 0.21 (10.7 PUFA divided by 50.3 S=0.21). In the preliminary 1970 report this ratio had risen to 0.41 (22.8 PUFA divided by 55.5 S=0.41). This change reflects an increase in the use of vegetable fats, i.e., margarine, shortening, salad and cooking oils. Friend states that "The per capita amount provided by animal fats has actually decreased because the large decreases in consumption of butter and lard were only partially offset by increases in fat associated with greater consumption of meat" and "Although calories from vegetable fats have increased from 5 to 16% since 1909-13, animal products still account for the largest share of the calories provided by fat."

Starch and sugar consumption have also changed. About equal proportions of starch and sugar are now consumed. In 1909-13 the ratio was two-thirds of calories from starch and one-third from sugar.

The Inter-Society Commission of Heart Disease Resources recommended (1970) limiting fat in the diet to less than 35% of total calories with less than 10% of the total calories from saturated fats. In the average American diet, 42.7% of the calories is from fat (Friend, 1971).

FAT-CONTROLLED DIETS

Guidelines to Planning and Nutrition Counseling

Observing the following concepts can implement a lifetime pattern of good nutrition for the patient and his family and may assist in keeping atherosclerosis risk factors low.

An approximately equal distribution of foods among the day's meals will promote good nutrition. The metabolic overload of an inordinately large amount of food or alcoholic beverage at one time should be avoided.

Maintenance of ideal weight is desirable. There is general acceptance of calorie control as a means to alleviate hypertension which carries a high atherosclerosis risk.

With a family history of atherosclerosis or diabetes, early medical consultation is advisable. Dietary moderation starting early in life is encouraged. Dietary restriction begun late in life is less effective in altering the undesirable course of events. With thorough dietary instruction long-term food habits can be developed around dietary changes to provide acceptable meals for the family.

Grain products, fruits, and vegetables should be the chief source of carbohydrate. Sugar and other sweets should be limited, and their use distributed among the day's meals. They should be used mainly as a flavoring ingredient in combined foods such as custards, puddings, and baked goods.

Refined sugars and alcohol are absorbed more rapidly than starches. Any excess over immediate tissue needs or glycogen storage capacity is converted to fat for storage in body tissues. Starches and other polysaccharides require breakdown before sugars from their digestion can be absorbed. This process is slower than that of the sugars; they are less apt to contribute to lipogenesis or to high serum triglycerides.

Moderation in the use of fats is recommended. This requires selection of lean meat and restriction of foods containing animal fats. Such restriction of saturated fat intake will assist in reducing cholesterol consumption to below 300 mg per day as recommended by the Inter-Society Commission for Heart Disease Resources (1970) and will help control calories.

A program of daily exercise should be promoted, smoking discouraged and moderation in the use of salt and alcohol recommended.

REFERENCES

Metabolism

Coleman, JE: Metabolic interrelationships between carbohydrates, lipids, and proteins. In Bondy, PK; Rosenberg, LE (Eds.): *Duncan's Diseases of Metabolism,* 6th ed. Philadelphia, Saunders, 1969. Genetics and Metabolism, Chap V.

Dietschy, JM; Wilson, JD: Regulation of cholesterol metabolism. *N Engl J Med, 282*:1128, 1179, 1241, 1970.

————; Weis, HJ: Cholesterol synthesis by gastrointestinal tract. *Am J Clin Nutr, 24*:70, 1971.

Friend, B: *Nutritional review. National Food Situation.* NFS-134, USDA, Washington, DC, 1970, and NFS-138, 1971.

Grundy, SM; Ahrens, EH, Jr: The effects of unsaturated fats on absorption, excretion, synthesis, and distribution of cholesterol in man. *J Clin Invest, 49*:1135, 1970.

Harris, PL; Embree, ND: Quantitative considerations of the effect of polyunsaturated fatty acid content of the diet upon the requirements for vitamin E. *Am J Clin Nutr, 13*:385, 1963.

Henry, JB: Clinical chemistry—lipids. In Davidsohn, I; Henry, JB (Eds.): *Todd-Sanford Clinical Diagnosis,* 14th ed. Philadelphia, Saunders, 1969.

Herman, RH; Zakim, D; Stifel, FB: Effect of diet on lipid metabolism in experimental animals and man. *Fed Proc, 29*:1302, 1970.

Holman, R: Biological activities of and requirements for polyunsaturated fatty acids. In *Progress in Chemistry of Fats and Other Lipids IX* (Part 5). New York, Pergamon Press, 1970.

Keys, A: Blood lipids in man—a brief review. *J Am Diet Assoc, 51*:508, 1967.

Nestel, PJ; Carol, KF; Havenstein, N: Plasma triglyceride response to carbohydrates, fats, and caloric intake. *Metabolism, 19*:1, 1970.

Pinckney, ER: The biological toxicity of polyunsaturated fats. *Medical Counterpoint, 5*:53, February 1973.

Regional Medical Program Service and American Heart Association: Report of the Inter-Society Commission for Heart Disease Resources: Primary prevention of atherosclerotic diseases. *Circulation, 42*:A55, 1970.

Ruderman, NB; Toews, CJ; Shafrir, E: The role of free fatty acids in glucose homeostasis. *Arch Intern Med, 123*:299, 1969.

Senior, JR (Ed.): *Medium Chain Triglycerides.* Philadelphia, Univ of Pennsylvania Press, 1968.

Wilson, FA; Dietschy, JM: Differential diagnostic approach to clinical problems of malabsorption. *Gastroenterology, 61*:911, 1971. (Mechanisms of fat absorption, and information on the pathophysiology of various disorders of fat absorption.)

Hyperlipoproteinemia

Arteriosclerosis: Report by NHLI Task Force on Arteriosclerosis, Vol. II. DHEW Publ no (NIH) 72-219. Washington, DC, US Govt Printing Office, 1971.

Fredrickson, DS, et al: *Dietary Management of Hyperlipoproteinemia:A Handbook for Physicians,* revised. Bethesda, Natl Heart and Lung Inst, 1971.

————; Levy, RI; Lees, RS: Fat transport of lipoproteins; an integrated approach to mechanisms and disorders. *N Engl J Med, 276*:34, 94, 148, 215, 273, 1967.

Kritchevsky, D: Normal regulation of blood lipid levels. *Mod Treat, 6*: 1302, 1969.

Lees, RS; Wilson, DE: The treatment of hyperlipidemia. *N Engl J Med, 284*:186, 1971.

Levy, RI; Bonnell, M; Ernst, ND: Dietary management of hyperlipoproteinemia. *J Am Diet Assoc, 58*:406, 1971.

————; Fredrickson, DS: Diagnosis and management of hyperlipoproteinemia. *Am J Cardiol, 22*:576, 1968.

————; Langer, T: Mechanisms involved in hyperlipidemia. *Mod Treat, 6*:1313, 1969.

————, et al: Dietary and drug treatment of primary hyperlipoproteinemia. *Ann Intern Med, 77*:267, 1972.

Quintao, E; Grundy, SM; Ahrens, EH, Jr: Effects of dietary cholesterol on the total body cholesterol in man. *J Lipid Res, 12*:233, 1971.

Stanbury, JB; Wyngaarden, JB; Fredrickson, DS (Eds.): *The Metabolic Basis of Inherited Disease,* 3rd ed. New York, McGraw Hill, 1972.

Dietary Planning and Food Composition

American Heart Association, American Dietetic Association, Heart Disease Control Program, and US Public Health Service: *Planning Fat-Controlled Meals for 1200 and 1800 Calories,* revised. New York, Am Heart A, 1966.

————: *Planning Fat-Controlled Meals for Approximately 2000 to 2600 Calories,* revised. New York, Am Heart Assoc, 1967.

Anderson, DB, et al: Effect of cooking on fatty acid composition of beef lipids. *J Fd Technol, 6*:141, 1971.

Bowman, F: MCT cookies, cakes and quick breads: Quality and acceptability. *J Am Diet Assoc, 62*:180, 1973.

Brown, HB: Food patterns that lower blood lipids in man. *J Am Diet Assoc, 58*:303, 1971.

Criner, PE; Feeley, RM: Evaluating analytical data on cholesterol in foods. *J Am Diet Assoc, 61*:115, 1972.

Feeley, RM; Criner, PE, and Watt, BK: Cholesterol content of foods. *J Am Diet Assoc, 61*:134, 1972.

Fletcher, ES; Foster, N; Anderson, JT; Grande, F; Keys, A: Quantitative estimation of diets to control serum cholesterol. *Am J Clin Nutr, 20*: 475, 1967.

Howard, B; Morse, E: Muffins and pastry made with medium chain triglyceride oil. *J Am Diet Assoc, 62*:51, 1973.

McIntire, JM: New dairy and related products. *Am J Public Health, 61*: 157, 1971.

Miljanich, P; Ostwald, R: Fatty acids in the newer brands of margarines. *J Am Diet Assoc, 56*:29, 1970.

Monsen, ER; Andriaenssens, L: Fatty acid composition and total lipid of cream and cream substitutes. *Am J Clin Nutr, 22*:458, 1969.

Monsen, ER; Crawford, PB; Lowe, DW: Diet margarines: Fat content, serving portions and acceptance. *J Am Diet Assoc, 54*:29, 1969.

Schizas, AA, et al: Medium-chain triglycerides: Use in food preparation. *J Am Diet Assoc, 51*:228, 1967.

Standal, BR, et al: Fatty acids, cholesterol, and proximate analyses of some ready-to-eat foods. *J Am Diet Assoc, 56*:392, 1970.

Zukel, M: Revising booklets on fat-controlled meals. *J Am Diet Assoc, 54*:20, 1969.

MODIFICATIONS IN CONSTITUENTS: C. CARBOHYDRATE

DIETS RESTRICTED IN LACTOSE

Rationale

L ACTASE DEFICIENCY OF EITHER genetic origin or secondary to mucosal damage by acute infection has been implicated as a cause of chronic gastrointestinal symptoms such as increased gastric motility, abdominal cramps, flatulence, and diarrhea. The enzyme lactase is essential for the digestion of lactose, a double sugar found in milk. Production of the enzyme may be totally lacking or merely deficient in quantity.

The objective of treatment is to prevent the above symptoms with the least dietary restriction possible.

Diet Plan

These diets follow the daily food guide (Section I) except that milk and other products that contain lactose are either eliminated or restricted to the individual's tolerance level. Lactose, generally referred to as milk sugar, is in the serum (or watery part) of milk. In making cheese most of the lactose is removed by draining off the whey and washing the curd. Within a month the small amount which remains is hydrolyzed to glucose and galactose by the bacteria present. As aging continues the glucose is used first by the bacteria, then the galactose, so that aged cheese is practically free of lactose (Fagen, et al., 1952). The curd of cottage cheese is also washed to remove whey and is therefore lower in lactose content than the milk from which it is made.

Fermented milks such as yogurt and buttermilk vary widely in lactose content depending upon the degree of acidity present to hydrolyze the lactose to glucose and galactose. Holtzman (1970) states that fermented milks generally are tolerated and can serve as a source of calcium.

Lactose-Free Test Diet

When clinical symptoms indicate the need to study lactose intolerance as a causative factor, a lactose-free diet may be used for a relatively short time. In this diet neither milk nor milk-containing foods would be used, not even butter and margarine, which has less than one percent lactose content. With this marked restriction the diet will be marginal or deficient in a number of nutrients unless special precautions are taken. See the calculated nutrient estimates for these diets in this section. Calcium, iron, and vitamins may need to be supplied.

Foods included in this diet are:
Meats, fish, poultry; eggs. Meat-base formulas for infants.
Dry beans and peas; nuts, peanut butter without milk solids.
Soy milk and soy milk infant formulas.
Cereals, flour, pastas.
Oils, lard, vegetable shortenings.
Vegetables, fruits, and their juices.
Sugars, jellies, fruit preserves.
Non-dairy whipped toppings and coffee whiteners if lactose-free. These products contain corn syrup solids and vegetable fats but not always lactose. However, *some may contain lactose*. Most of them contain a milk protein (McIntire, 1971) which is allowed on the diet.

Persons buying food for this diet should read the labels and avoid those products containing milk. All of the carbohydrate of milk is lactose.

Restricted Lactose Diets

Short Term Liquid Diet

When a person has severe symptoms of lactose malabsorption and cannot tolerate a general diet, a liquid diet limited to 5 grams of lactose is indicated. One-half cup of half-and-half (12% cream) contains this quantity and may be added to the foods listed for the lactose-free test diet. Six feedings a day are recommended. Breakfast cereals may be made into gruels with fruit juice or water;

vegetables and meats pureed after cooking and combined with broth; and pureed fruit and fruit juices gelled for a change in consistency. Instead of one-half cup of 12 percent cream, other foods in the quantities to provide 5 gm lactose may be selected from Table VI-22, *Lactose in Portions of Some Foods,* in this section. When symptoms subside a more general diet in respect to consistency and lactose content may be used.

TABLE VI-22
LACTOSE CONTENT OF PORTIONS OF SOME FOODS

Food	Portion	Lactose gm
Butter	1 teaspoon (1/5 oz)	0.02
Cheddar cheese	1 ounce	0.60*
Cottage cheese, creamed	1/2 cup	3.50
Cream, coffee (20%)	2 tablespoons (1 oz)	1.30
Half-and-half (12%)	2 tablespoons (1 oz)	1.30
Margarine	1 teaspoon (1/5 oz)	0.02
Milk, whole	1 cup	12.00
Milk, 2% with added milk solids	1 cup	15.00
Milk, skim	1 cup	12.00

*Less for well-aged cheese.

Restricted Lactose General Diet

Absence of symptoms is the criterion for adjusting the level of lactose in the diet to the individual's tolerance by the addition of measured amounts of lactose-containing foods. These are added to a lactose-free diet in graded steps of 10 gm lactose each. According to Bayless and Huang (1969) tolerance for lactose is highly individual. It may be only 25 to 30 gm for some; others may tolerate as high as 50 to 100 gm in a day. Dietary progression is at the direction of the physician.

It is important that the lactose-containing food be eaten with a meal and not all at one time.

In planning the restricted lactose general diet, foods for a three-meal-a-day plan are selected from those listed in the lactose-free test diet, and lactose-containing foods are added gradually as tolerance permits. With poor absorption and milk restriction, this diet generally needs mineral and vitamin supplementation, with emphasis on calcium, iron, magnesium, riboflavin, vitamin B_6, B_{12}, and folic acid. See Table I-3, page 25, for nutrients needed to compensate for removal of milk from the diet.

The restricted lactose general diet used as a basis for calcula-

TABLE VI-23

CALCULATED NUTRIENT ESTIMATES OF LACTOSE-RESTRICTED DIETS
AS SERVED IN A HOSPITAL

Nutrients	Unit	Man 23-50 years old	Woman 23-50 years old	Lactose-free test diet	Restricted lactose liquid diet	Restricted lactose general diet
Food energy	Kcal	2,700	2,000	1,694	1,180	2,189
Protein	gm	56	46	90	35	102
Fat	gm	—	—	46	25	80
Carbohydrate	gm	—	—	238	205	272
Lactose	gm				5	25
Calcium	gm	0.8	0.8	0.3	0.3	1.0
Phosphorus	gm	0.8	0.8	1.2	0.5	1.5
Iron	mg	10.0	18.0	17.6	8.0	17.2
Magnesium	mg	350	300	327	176	333
Sodium	mg	—	—	3,235	1,852	3,641
Sodium mEq				141	80	158
Potassium	mg	—	—	2,714	2,022	3,276
Potassium mEq			—	6,836	2,907	7,961
Vitamin A	IU	5,000	4,000	70	52	94
Vitamin E		15 IU	12 IU	6 mg	2.5 mg	8.0 mg
Ascorbic acid	mg	45.0	45.0	92.0	167	96.0
Folacin	mg	0.4	0.4	—	—	—
Niacin equiv.	mg	18.0	13.0	34.5	16.0	35.9
Riboflavin	mg	1.6	1.2	1.3	0.7	2.2
Thimain	mg	1.4	1.0	1.7	0.6	1.9
Vitamin B$_6$	mg	2.0	2.0	2.0	1.2	2.1
Vitamin B$_{12}$	mcg	3.0	3.0	3.7	.9	5.3

tions of nutrient estimates includes 2 cups of milk and 3 pats of butter (72 cuts per pound) and provides about 25 gm lactose.

Foods to Avoid in Lactose-Restricted Diets

Avoid all milk and cheese products, and foods made with milk or cheese unless the lactose content is known and included in the day's allowance.

Avoid the following foods because of their variable or unknown lactose content. If the processor's formula is known a food may be calculated as part of the lactose allowance.

1. All baked foods unless especially prepared to eliminate milk products.
2. All breads except French and Italian. These are milk-free.
3. Canned and frozen vegetables prepared with sauce.
4. Cold meats and other sausage products.
5. Commercially breaded meats, fish, poultry.
6. Cooked milk-base salad dressings. French dressing and mayonnaise are standardized products made without milk.

7. Dehydrated potatoes unless prepared without milk. Read the label.
8. Milk chocolate and candies made with milk solids and/or butter. (Hard candies may be used.)
9. Prepared mixes and puddings of all kinds.
10. Soups made with milk, cheese, butter, margarine.

DIET RESTRICTED IN GALACTOSE

Rationale

Galactosemia results from a hereditary lack of an enzyme that is essential for the conversion of galactose to glucose for use by the body. Lactose is hydrolyzed to galactose and glucose in the intestine, In the absence of this enzyme there is an accumulation of galactose in the red cells of the blood.

Diet Plan

A galactose-free diet may be selected from the foods listed for use in the foregoing lactose-free diet with these reservations:

Stachyose, a tetrasaccharide, is present in beets, peas, lima beans, and in soybeans and soy products. It is thought by some that stachyose is a source of galactose (Robinson, 1967). Meat-base formulas are available for use instead of soy products for infants that require a galactose-free diet.

Liver, brains, and pancreas store galactose and may also be a source, so are excluded from the diet.

Nutrient supplementation needs will be the same as for the low lactose diet.

REFERENCES

Alpers, DH; Isselbacher, KJ: Disaccharidase deficiency. *Adv Metab Disord,* 4:75, 1970.

Bayless, TM; Huang, S: Inadequate intestinal digestion of lactose. *Am J Clin Nutr,* 22:250, 1969.

Brown, CH: *Diagnostic Procedures in Gastroenterology.* St. Louis, Mosby, 1967.

Dahlquist, A: Disaccharide intolerance. *JAMA, 195*:225, 1966.

Dunphy, JV et al: Intestinal lactase deficit in adults. *Gastroenterology, 49*: 12, 1965.

Fagen, HJ; Stine, JB; Hussong, RV: The identification of reducing sugars in cheddar cheese during the early stages of ripening. *J Dairy Sci, 35*: 779, 1952.

Flock, MH: Recent contributions in intestinal absorption and malabsorption. A review. *Am J Clin Nutr, 20*:327, 1969.

Gray, GM: Intestinal digestion and maldigestion of carbohydrates. *Annu Rev Med, 23*:391, 1971.

Holtzman, NA: Dietary treatment of inborn errors of metabolism. *Annu Rev Med, 21*:335, 1970.

McGill, DB; Newcomer, AD: Primary and secondary disaccharidase deficiencies. *Prog in Gastroenterology, 2*:22, 1970.

McIntire, JM: New dairy and related products. *Am J Public Health, 61*: 157, 1969.

Robinson, CH: *Proud fit-Robinson's Normal and Therapeutic Nutrition,* New York, Macmillan, 1967.

Rosensweig, NS: Adult human milk intolerance and intestinal lactase deficiency. A review. *J Dairy Sci, 52*:585, 1969.

Weser, E; Jeffries, GH; Sleisinger, MH: Malabsorption. *Gastroenterology, 50*:811, 1966.

Galactosemia

Hansen, RG: Hereditary galactosemia. *JAMA, 208*:2077, 1969.

Hsia, DYY (Ed.): *Galactosemia.* Springfield, Thomas, 1969.

Wong, PWK; Hsai, DYY: Inborn errors of metabolism. In Goodhart, RS; Shils, ME (Eds.): *Modern Nutrition in Health and Disease,* 5th ed. Philadelphia, Lea and Febiger, 1973.

MODIFICATIONS IN CONSTITUENTS:
D. DIETS CONTROLLED IN
PROTEIN, FAT, AND CARBOHYDRATE

DIET IN DIABETES MELLITUS

THE COMMITTEE ON FOOD AND NUTRITION of the American Diabetes Association observes that the nutritional requirements of the person with diabetes are basically the same as for the non-diabetic; the nutrient recommendations of the National Research Council provide acceptable levels in planning (Bierman, et al, 1971). The following are the Committee's recommendations:

1. The single most important objective in the nutritional care of persons with diabetes mellitus is to achieve and maintain ideal body weight.
2. The same proportion of carbohydrates as in the general consumption level (1971) in the United States, 45 percent of the calories of the diet, is a satisfactory level. Liberalization of the carbohydrate for the person with diabetes will have the desirable effect of providing a reciprocal decrease in fats and cholesterol. However persons with hypertriglyceridemia may require a lower carbohydrate intake since triglyceride serum levels are sensitive to increases in dietary carbohydrate. The dietary prescription should reflect the laboratory findings as to serum lipoproteins.
3. Risk factors associated with premature and accelerated atherosclerosis (for example: obesity, hyperglycemia and hyperlipidemia) should be kept to a minimum. Reduction of serum lipids can be achieved by limiting calories, saturated fat, and cholesterol in the diet. Use of appropriate drugs may be warranted for certain types of hyperlipoproteinemia; insulin or oral hypergylcemic agents may be needed in the treatment of diabetes mellitus.
4. A general health program for the individual should include peri-

odic health examinations, regular exercise, avoidance of cigarette smoking, attention to personal hygiene and prevention of infection.

5. Food intake should be regular and spaced in relation to the type and time of insulin administration and physical activity. Periods of "feast and fast" should be avoided. Food for the day for persons with diabetes is usually divided into 4 feedings (Table VI-24. Five may be required for some individuals.

6. Rapid and/or excessive ingestion of soluble sugars and alcohol should be avoided.

Diet Plan

Basic recommendations for planning diets for individuals with diabetes are these:

1. Calories adjusted to achieve and maintain ideal weight. Maintenance diets should meet the minimum level for various body weights and ages (NAS-NRC Recommended Dietary Allowances, 1973).

2. Approximately 45% of the diet from carbohydrate. Concentrated carbohydrates are not used except in very limited quantities.

3. Fat controlled at about 1 gram per kilogram of ideal body weight. This will maintain a relatively low fat content in the diet. To follow the American Heart Association recommendations for average individuals, cholesterol content of the day's food should not be over 300 mg. Use of lean meat and skim milk will do much to meet these requirements. Use of all-vegetable fat margarines will further reduce the saturated fat and cholesterol levels in the diet.

4. One gram protein per kilogram body weight has been recommended. If the percentage of fat and/or carbohydrate are decreased, protein will be reciprocally increased. Cost of the diet will also be increased.

5. Each meal of the day including between-meal nourishments should include some protein, fat, and carbohydrate. Distribution of these nutrients throughout the day will help maintain the blood sugar within an even range. Although food selection within the food groups will vary from day to day, the level of intake of protein, fat, and carbohydrate should remain relatively constant. Broadening the exchange items within the bread-cereal group can provide greater variety to the diet at a relatively uniform level of intake.

Within the requirements of the physician's prescription, a dietary regimen should be planned in consultation with the patient and his family to insure that it is adapted to his abilities, resources, and social needs. Making the individual a partner in organizing a nutrition program adapted to him will assist in developing a sense of commitment, personal responsibility, and independence in the dietary control of his diabetes.

The diet should be reviewed periodically by the physician and adjustments made as indicated by the patient's medical and social history. During counseling sessions, emphasis can be given to the selection within the exchange groups of foods of high nutritional value, particularly the milk, whole grain breads, cereals, dark green and deep yellow vegetables, and fruits high in vitamin C.

Focusing on some of the problems the individual is encountering in following his diet will often reveal economic and social needs which require adjustments in the meal pattern. Counseling sessions provide an opportunity to again emphasize to the patient that "special" foods are not necessary and to warn him against some of the high priced "health foods." The nutrition counselor can do much to help the patient understand that his diet plan is a good nutrition pattern for the entire family. The dietitian's role is to provide support to the patient in learning to manage his diet, in appreciating and accepting the many requirements for a lifetime maintenance of health program, and in achieving independence and dignity in meeting his personal needs.

Food intake is critical for the individual with diabetes. It is desirable to maintain approximately the same diet from day to day, with carbohydrate, protein, and fat distributed over all the meals. Variety can be achieved by use of the food exchange system. To avoid hypoglycemia, a person receiving insulin or other hypoglycemic agent may need a suitable replacement if he cannot eat an appreciable portion of his regular diet. This is usually done by selecting a higher carbohydrate food, either liquid or solid, and replacing on a glucose equivalent basis. Glucose is formed in the metabolism of foods in the following ratios:

> 100 percent of carbohydrate
> 58 percent of protein (For rapid calculation,
> > 50 percent is frequently used.)
> 10 percent of fat
> Total = glucose equivalent value of food.

In case of insulin reaction, food providing 5 to 10 grams of rapidly available glucose is usually given. A teaspoon of sugar will supply about 5 grams available glucose. One half cup of orange juice is counted as 10 grams available glucose, one half cup milk as 9 grams. The milk which contains protein, fat, and carbohydrate will be absorbed more slowly than the sugar or orange juice.

During periods of illness when food is not well tolerated a soft or liquid diet may be necessary. It is desirable to include some protein in these plans. Milk, eggs, plain tender meats, toast, bread, and cereals are generally well tolerated. In case of nausea, Marble, et al (1971) recommended 3 to 4 ounces of liquid food containing carbohydrate every hour or two. However, following vomiting, delaying ingestion two to three hours may avoid a recurrence. Replacement of electrolytes is important.

Table VI-24 Meal Pattern: 1800 Calorie Diet, Diabetes Mellitus

Food Group		Protein gm	Fat gm	Carbohydrate gm	Calories	Cholesterol mg
Breakfast						
Fruit	1 exchange	0	0	10	40	0
Cereal	1 exchange	2	0	15	70	0
Meat group	1 exchange	7	5	0	75	25
Bread	1 exchange	2	0	15	70	0
Fat	2 exchanges	0	10	0	90	*
Milk, skim	1 exchange	8	—	12	80	7
		19	15	52	425	32
Noon						
Meat group	2 exchanges	14	10	0	150	50
Bread	2 exchanges	4	0	30	140	0
A vegetable	No limit			Negligible		0
Fruit	2 exchanges	0	0	20	80	0
Fat	2 exchanges	0	10	0	90	*
		18	20	50	460	50
Evening						
Meat group	3 exchanges	21	15	0	225	75
A vegetable	No limit			Negligible		
B vegetable	2 exchanges	4	0	14	70	0
Fruit	2 exchanges	0	0	20	80	0
Fat	2 exchanges	0	10	0	90	*
		25	25	34	465	75
Night						
Meat group	2 exchanges	14	10	0	150	50
Bread	2 exchanges	4	0	30	140	0
Fat	1 exchange	0	5	0	45	
Fruit	1 exchange	0	0	10	40	0
Milk, skim	1 exchange	8	—	12	80	7
		26	15	52	455	57
Totals and calorie distribution		88 (20%)	75 (38%)	188 (42%)	1805	214

*All vegetable margarine and vegetable oils used are cholesterol free. Butter = 12 mg cholesterol per exchange. See Table VI-14 Cholesterol Exchanges for other cholesterol values.

Before going home, the patient as well as family should have written instructions on how to select foods when eating out, foods for picnics and parties, foods for travel and foods for periods of illness. The need for exercise should be appreciated as well as good hygiene and dental care. The community resources should be known and encouragement should be given to telephone the dietitian or public health nurse if in doubt. They in turn will refer the patient to the physician as warranted.

Several of the references at the end of this section give detailed examples of soft and liquid diets and diabetic diets modified for other disease conditions. Suitable between-meal nourishments are discussed. List of further sources of information on exchange values of combined foods (soups, entrées, etc) is included in the references.

In the meal pattern for the 1800 calorie diet (Table VI-24) the cholesterol content of the diet is calculated without egg. Three eggs per week would provide an average of 118 mg cholesterol daily.

Cholesterol content of diet is based on use of all-vegetable margarines. Use of butter would add 12 mg cholesterol per teaspoon.

The distribution of calories is comparable in this diet to the hospital general diet and to the diets controlled in fat.

REFERENCES

Bierman, EL, et al: Principles of nutrition and dietary recommendations for patients with diabetes mellitus: 1971. *Diabetes, 20:*633, 1971.

Cahill, GF, et al: Practical developments in diabetes research. In Proceedings of the Fiftieth Anniversary Insulin Symposium. Indianapolis, Indiana, October 18-20, 1971. *Diabetes, 21,* (Suppl 2):703, 1972.

Diabetes Mellitus, 7th ed, revised. Indianapolis, Indiana, Lilly Research Laboratories, 1970.

Felig, P; Bondy, PK (Guest Eds.): Symposium on diabetes mellitus. *Med Clin North Am, 55:*790, 1971.

Friedman, GJ: Diet in the treatment of diabetes mellitus. In Goodhart, RS; Shils, ME (Eds.): *Modern Nutrition in Health and Disease.* Philadelphia, Lea and Febiger, 1973, Chap 29.

Gormican, A: *Controlling Diabetes with Diet.* Springfield, Thomas, 1971.

Meal Planning with Exchange Lists, revised. Prepared by Committees of American Diabetes Association, Inc, American Dietetic Association in cooperation with the Chronic Disease Program, Public Health Service, HEW, 1956.

Marble, A; White, P; Bradley, RF; Krall, LP (Eds.): *Joslin's Diabetes Mellitus.* Philadelphia, Lea and Febiger, 1971.

Revell, DT: *Gourmet Recipes for Diabetics: An International Diabetic Diet Book.* Springfield, Thomas, 1971.
Sussman, KE (Ed.): *Juvenile-Type Diabetes and Its Complications.* Springfield, Thomas, 1971.
Traisman, HS: *Management of Juvenile Diabetes Mellitus,* 2nd ed. St. Louis, Mosby, 1971.

KETOGENIC DIET

Although drugs have largely replaced diet in the treatment of epilepsy in children, a ketogenic diet is tried occasionally. This diet reverses the usual ratio of fat to carbohydrate. This means that carbohydrate must be severely restricted and fats markedly increased. The objective is to furnish an insufficient quantity of glucose so that complete metabolic breakdown of fats cannot take place and acetone bodies (acetone, aceto-acetic acid, and beta-hydroxy butyric acid) will accumulate to produce ketosis.

Diet Plans

An allowance of 1.0 to 1.5 grams of protein per kilogram of body weight is maintained. This quantity can be increased if the person likes meat. Ketogenic factors (fatty acids) are derived from 90 percent of the fat and about 50 percent of the protein; anti-ketogenic factors (glucose as an end product) include 100 percent of the carbohydrate, 10 percent of the fat, and approximately 50 percent of the protein.

Quick dietary calculations which approximate the desired ratio are based on the dietary unit derived from the ketogenic: anti-ketogenic ratio (fatty acid to available glucose). The diet is constructed as follows:

Calories: As prescribed according to NAS-NRC recommended dietary allowance.
Protein: As prescribed; generally 1.0 to 1.5 gm per kg of body weight.
Fat and carbohydrate are calculated from a dietary unit based on the desired ratio which may be a ratio from a 2 to 1 (fat to available glucose) to a 3 to 1 ratio. The 3 to 1 ratio is so restricted in carbohydrate foods that it is not practical except in emergency situations.

2:1 Ratio

One unit of a 2:1 diet contains 2 gms fat × 9 Kcal/gm = 18 Kcal
1 gm carbohydrate × 4 Kcal/gm = 4 Kcal

Dietary unit = 22 Kcal

Total calories desired divided by 22 gives the number of units used to determine the grams of fat and carbohydrate in the diet.

For a child eight to ten years old, a 2 to 1 ratio would be calculated as follows (This prescription does not conform to RDA.):

Dietary prescription: 2200 calories, 40 gms protein
Units in diet: 2200 divided by 22 (Kcal per unit) = 100 units
Fat: 100 units × 2 (prescribed ratio) = 200 gms   1800 calories
Protein: 40 gms   160 calories
Carbohydrate: (100 units minus
           40 grams protein)   =   60 gms   240 calories

                                              2200 calories
Calorie distribution: 82% fat, 7% protein, 11% carbohydrate

Food Allowance for Day
2 to 1 Ratio for 8 to 10 Year Old Child

Food	Amount	Protein gm	Fat gm	Carbohydrate gm
Egg	One	6.0	6.0	0
Meat, fish, poultry	3 exch.	21.0	15.0	0
Vegetables, 6% carbohydrate or less	2 cups	6.8	0	16.8
Bread exchange	1 slice	2.0	0	15.0
Orange juice (½ cup)	4 ounces	0.8	0	12.4
Fat exchanges	3 tablespoons	0	45.0	0
Whipping cream (1½ cups, 38% fat)	12 ounces	7.5	135.0	10.5
Totals		44.1	201.0	54.7

Food Allowance for Day
3 to 1 Ratio for 8 to 10 Year Old Child

Food	Amount	Protein gm	Fat gm	Carbohydrate gm
Egg	One	6.0	6.0	0
Meat, fish, poultry	3 exch.	21.0	15.0	0
Vegetables, 6% carbohydrate or less	1½ cups	5.1	0	12.6
Orange juice (¼ cup)	2 ounces	0.4	0	6.2
Fat exchanges	4 tablespoons	0	60	0
Whipping cream (1½ cups, 38% fat)	12 ounces	7.5	135.0	10.5
Totals		40.0	216.0	29.3

3:1 Ratio

For the same child, a 3 to 1 ratio would be calculated as follows:

One unit: 3 gms fat × 9 Kcal/gm   = 27 Kcal
         1 gm carbohydrate × 4 Kcal/gm   =   4 Kcal

                             Dietary unit   = 31 Kcal
Units in diet: 2200 calories divided by 31 (Kcal per unit) = 71 units

Fat: 71 units × 3 (prescribed ratio)   = 213 gms   1917 calories
Protein: = 40 gms   160 calories
Carbohydrate:
   (71 units minus 40 grams protein) = 31 gms   124 calories

                                        2201 calories
Calorie distribution: 87% fat, 7% protein, 6% carbohydrate

Management of the Ketogenic Diet

Mike (1965) recommended that the day's food be divided equally among three meals and served at regular times each day. No medications are to be taken except on a physician's prescription. Any preparations containing alcohol, sorbitol, mannitol, hexitol, or sugar will upset the balance of the diet.

This diet will not meet recommended allowances for several vitamins and minerals. Robinson (1972) recommends supplementation with calcium gluconate, 7.0 to 10.0 mg of iron, and a multivitamin preparation.

With restriction of the amount of vegetable and cereal products in the diet attention must be directed to providing adequate amounts of vitamin E in relation to the polyunsaturated fats included. See Appendix I, Vitamin E, for information on relationship of different vegetable oils to vitamin E deficiency.

Any vegetable with 6 percent or less of carbohydrate content can be used in the amount allowed in the diet plan. This will include all green leafy vegetables (spinach, beet greens, etc), asparagus, green and wax beans, cabbage, cauliflower, celery, cucumbers, eggplant, peppers, radishes, summer squash, tomatoes, tomato juice, and cooked white turnips. Fresh, canned, or frozen products may be used. One serving is considered to be one-half cup, 3-1/2 ounces, or 100 gms. Without weighting for frequency of use these vegetables average 1.7 gm protein, and 4.2 gm carbohydrate per 100 grams.

Signore (1973) describes research in progress on the use of diets using medium chain triglycerides and up to 19% of the calories from carbohydrates.

REFERENCES

Lasser, JI; Brush, MK: An improved ketogenic diet for the treatment of epilepsy. *J Am Diet Assoc, 62*:281, 1973.

Mike, EM: Practical guide and dietary management of children with seizures using the ketogenic diet. *Am J Clin Nutr, 17*:399, 1965.

Robinson, CH: *Normal and Therapeutic Nutrition,* 14th ed. New York. Macmillan, 1972.

Signore, JM: The ketogenic diet containing medium chain triglycerides. *J Am Diet Assoc, 62*:285, 1973.

MODIFICATIONS IN CONSTITUENTS:
E. DIETS CONTROLLED IN SODIUM

Rationale

THE AMOUNT OF SODIUM ingested is of concern when a disease condition has altered the body's homeostatic processes which maintain the serum sodium at about a normal level.

Indications for Use

Diets restricted in sodium are used in the treatment of edema in a wide variety of conditions including congestive heart failure, hypertension, cirrhosis of the liver, toxemia of pregnancy, some kidney diseases, and after the administration of adreno-cortical steroids.

A diet restricted in calories and sodium is indicated for those patients who may need to lose weight as well as limit their sodium intake.

A diet with increased protein and restricted in sodium is especially useful for people with nephrosis and for those with cirrhosis of the liver when accompanied by ascites.

Iodine supplementation is advisable when diets are restricted to 1000 mg sodium or less are used.

Diet Plans

Diet plans restricting sodium intake to three levels are outlined. These diets will meet the needs of most patients, but any of the nutrient levels (sodium, protein, calories) should be changed to meet the special needs of individuals.

1. *500 mg sodium daily, 22 mEq.* Low sodium diet with no restriction in calories.

TABLE VI-25

VALUES FOR FOOD GROUPS IN RESTRICTED SODIUM DIETS

Primary consideration is given to the sodium content of foods in this table. Values for calories, protein, fat, and carbohydrate are the same as in the food exchange lists in Section One, and food groups are the same with the exception of vegetables and meats. Regular foods are those prepared with salt. Food values from *Handbook 8*, Watt and Merrill, 1963.

Food Group	Amount	Calories	Protein gm	Fat gm	Carbohydrate gm	Sodium mg	Sodium mEq
Milk							
Whole	1 cup	170	8	10	12	122	5.3
Skim	1 cup	80	8	—	12	127	5.5
Low sodium	1 cup	170	8	10	12	6	0.3
Vegetables, List 2A (Table VI-26)							
Low sodium	1/2 cup	Negligible				9	0.4
Moderate sodium	1/2 cup	Negligible				40	1.7
Vegetables, List 2B (Table VI-26)							
Low sodium	1/2 cup	35	2	0	7	9	0.4
Moderate sodium	1/2 cup	35	2	0	7	40	1.7
Fruit, fruit juices	1 exchange	40	0	0	10	2	0.1
Bread-Cereal Group							
Regular bread	1 slice	70	2	0	15	122	5.3
Starchy vegetables in Bread-Cereal group	1 exchange	70	2	0	15	5	0.2
Low sodium bread	1 slice	70	2	0	15	5	0.2

Food Group	Amount	Calories	Protein gm	Fat gm	Carbohydrate gm	Sodium mg	Sodium mEq
Low-sodium ready-to-eat cereals	1 exchange	70	2	0	15	2	0.1
Cereals, pastas no salt added. See following explanation	1/2 cup, cooked	70	2	0	15	Negligible	
Meat, fish, poultry	1 exchange	55	8	3	0	22	1.0
Egg, 8 to lb	One	75	6	6	0	61	2.7
Low sodium peanut butter*	2 tablespoons	200	10	17	4	6	0.3
Fats							
Regular butter or margarine	1 teaspoon	45	0	5	0	49	2.1
Low sodium butter	1 teaspoon	45	0	5	0	0	0
Oils, salad or cooking	1 teaspoon	45	0	5	0	0	0
Sweets							
Granulated or powdered sugar†	1 tablespoon	50	0	0	12	Trace	
Cane or maple syrup†	1 tablespoon	50	0	0	12	Trace	
Honey, jellies, preserves	1 tablespoon	50	0	0	12	Trace	

*Processor's analysis.
†Brown sugar, corn syrup, and molasses contain more sodium than these.

2. *1,000 mg sodium daily, 44 mEq.* Moderate sodium-restricted diet with no limitation in calories.
3. *1,000 mg sodium, 1,200 calories.* Moderates sodium-restricted diet, decreased calories.
4. *1,000 mg sodium, 120 gm protein.* Moderate sodium-restricted diet, increased protein.
5. *2,400-4,500 mg sodium daily, 104 to 196 mEq.* Mild sodium-restricted diet with no limitation in calories.

LOW SODIUM DIETS

The 500 mg sodium diet is the lowest level usually found acceptable, and is usually the lowest level necessary. The sodium may be reduced by over 200 mg daily by the substitution of low sodium milk for regular milk. Low sodium milk, however, is expensive, relatively unpalatable, and not well accepted by most people.

Diet Plan: 500 mg Sodium (22 mEq), no restrictions in calories

Food Group	Amount	Sodium mg	Sodium mEq
Milk, whole or skim	2 cups	244	10.6
Vegetables, low sodium only	4 exchanges	36	1.6
Fruit, fruit juices	3 exchanges	6	0.3
Low sodium bread	4 slices	22	1.0
Low sodium ready-to-eat cereals	1 exchange	1	0.1
Starchy vegetables listed in bread-cereal group	1 exchange	5	0.2
Cereals, pastas, cooked	As desired	Negligible	
Meat, poultry, fish (See Table VI-5*)	5 ounces	110	4.7
Eggs (3/7)	3/week	26	1.1
Total		450	19.6

Other foods of negligible sodium value may be used as desired. These include: Salt-free butter, margarine, salad dressings, oils, granulated or powdered sugar, jelly, honey, cane or maple syrup.

Diet Plan: 1,000 mg Sodium (44 mEq), no restriction in calories

The 1,000 mg sodium diet follows the same plan as the 500 mg

	Sodium mg	Sodium mEq
1/4 teaspoon table salt (1-1/2 grams)	580	25.2
1 serving-packet table salt (1 gram)	388	16.9
1 cup milk, whole or skim	122	5.3
3 slices regular bread, whole wheat, white, cracked wheat, American rye	366	15.9
3 teaspoons regular butter or margarine	148	6.4
1 egg, 8 to a lb.	61	2.7
1 exchange of a moderate sodium vegetable (see list)	40	1.7

sodium diet but adds 1/4 teaspoon table salt daily or its equivalent in foods. The amounts of sodium in table salt and in some foods are listed here so that a person may select a source of additional sodium that is most appealing to him.

Diet Plan: 1,000 mg Sodium (44 mEq), calories restricted to 1,200

			Sodium	
Food Group	*Amount*	*Calories*	*mg*	*mEq*
Milk, skim	2 cups	160	244	10.6
Vegetables:				
Low sodium, List 2A*	3 exchanges	Negligible	27	1.2
Moderate sodium, List 2B*	1 exchange	35	40	1.7
Fruit, unsweetened fruit juices	3 exchanges	120	6	0.3
Regular bread	3 slices	210	366	15.9
Starchy vegetables	1 exchange	70	5	0.2
or cooked cereals or pastas	[1/2 cup]	[70]	[Negligible]	
Low sodium ready-to-eat cereal	1 exchange	70	2	0.1
Meat, fish, poultry	6 ounces	330	132	5.7
Eggs (3/7)	3/week	34	26	1.1
Regular butter or margarine	3 teaspoons	135	148	6.4
Total		1,164	996	43.2

Diet Plan: 1,000 mg Sodium (44 mEq), Protein 120 grams

			Sodium	
Food Group	*Amount*	*Calories*	*mg*	*mEq*
Milk, whole or skim	5 cups	40	610	26.5
Vegetables:				
Low sodium, List 2A*	3 exchanges	Negligible	27	1.2
Moderate sodium, List 2B*	1 exchange	2	40	1.7
Fruit, fruit juices	3 exchanges	0	6	0.3
Low sodium bread	3 slices	6	15	0.7
Starchy vegetables†	2 exchanges	4	10	0.4
Low sodium ready-to-eat cereal	1 exchange	2	2	0.1
Meat, fish, poultry	8 ounces	64	176	7.7
Eggs (3/7)	3/week	3	26	1.1
Low sodium butter or margarine	As desired	0	0	0
Granulated or powdered sugar,				
jelly, honey, syrup	Allowed	0	0	0
Total		121	912	39.7

*See Table VI-26, Vegetables Grouped for Average Sodium Content, page 210.
†One cup cooked breakfast cereal or pasta may be substituted for the two exchanges of starchy vegetables.

Diet Plan: 2,400-4,500 mg Sodium (104-196 mEq)

The mild sodium-restricted diet allows an intake of from 2,400 to 4,500 mg sodium daily (104-196 mEq). To accomplish a diet within this range the following general plan is outlined:

1. Foods are lightly salted in preparation, using about one-half of

the amount that is customary. If the food already has salt added, as in the case of canned vegetables, no salt is added.

2. Milk is included at 2 cups a day for an adult.
3. Regular bread and butter or margarine are included.
4. Highly salted foods are not used. See list of foods to avoid in this section.

SODIUM IN FOODS

Milk Group

Whole or skim milk, the light table creams, and plain yogurt average about the same amount of sodium: 50 mg/100 gm or 122 mg (5.3 mEq) per cup. Chocolate drink, made with either whole or skim milk, contains slightly less sodium and may be used as an alternate. Partially skimmed milk with 2% milk solids added is higher in sodium than whole or skim milk; and cultured buttermilk is about 2-1/2 times as high. Neither of these are included in the low or moderate sodium diets.

Ice cream, ice milk, and sherbet (without added salt) may be used as follows: Two ounces of ice cream with 10 percent butterfat or of ice milk contain about 40 mg sodium (Watt and Merrill, 1963), and either may be an alternate for 1/3 cup milk in the 1,000 mg sodium diets.

Three ounces of orange sherbet contain about 9 mg sodium and may be an alternate for a low sodium vegetable in the restricted sodium but not in the restricted calorie diets.

Vegetables

Table VI-26 includes vegetables that are raw, cooked, canned without added salt (dietary pack), or frozen without processing brine treatment. Some of the sodium content of the vegetables is leached out in cooking or canning and is contained in the liquid. This accounts for the difference between the listed raw and cooked items. Values are for drained solids.

Softened water should not be used in food preparation.

For convenience in dietary calculations vegetables are grouped in the table according to sodium content, and the food exchange system.

	Sodium Content		
	Range	*Average*	*mEq*
Low sodium	1 mg to 25 mg/100 gm	9 mg/100 gm	0.4
Moderate sodium	25 mg to 50 mg/100 gm	40 mg/100 gm	1.7
High sodium	75 mg to 159 mg/100 gm	—	—

Most vegetables are in the low sodium group and in List 2A of the food exchange system, but some of List 2A and several of List 2B contain sodium in the 25 to 50 mg/100 gm range.

Starchy vegetables, included as exchanges in Table VI-26 average 5 mg sodium per serving. The size of an average serving for all groups is 100 gm (3 1/2 ounces) or about 1/2 cup.

Frozen vegetables vary in the method of preparation. Some have added salt; some have monosodium glutamate. Read the labels. Those that do not have salt or monosodium glutamate added may be used according to the table. Frozen peas and lima beans are processed by a brine flotation method which adds sodium. They are usually not included in a sodium-restricted diet.

Vegetables that are pickled (cucumbers) or brined (sauerkraut) are not included in any of the sodium-restricted diets. Hominy (lye treated) is not included. Vegetable juices (except tomato juice processed without salt) should not be used.

Small amounts (1 ounce or less) of any of the low sodium vegetables may be used without being counted in the 500 or 1,000 mg sodium diets. One such addition may be made in a day.

Small amounts (1 ounce or less) of any of the moderate sodium vegetables may be used and counted as a 9-mg sodium exchange.

If any of the high sodium vegetables are used in small amounts (1 ounce or less) they must be counted as an exchange of a moderate sodium vegetable (40 mg sodium).

Diets planned for 500 mg sodium are limited to low sodium vegetables and to small amounts of moderate sodium vegetables as an occasional alternate for an exchange of a low sodium one.

Diets planned for 1,000 mg sodium may occasionally include a small amount (1 ounce or less) of a high sodium vegetable as an alternate for an exchange of a moderate sodium vegetable.

Fruit

Raw fruits, in the quantities listed as fruit exchanges in Section I, are included in restricted sodium diets at 2 mg sodium each. Fruit canned without sugar is counted at the same sodium and calorie values. Fruit listed in the 1,200 calorie diet is limited to these two kinds.

Fruit canned with sugar and fruit sweetened and frozen are

TABLE VI-26

VEGETABLES GROUPED FOR AVERAGE SODIUM CONTENT

Raw or Cooked; or only as noted

Low Sodium Average: 9 mg Sodium Per Serving Range: 1-25 mg per 100 gm	Moderate Sodium Average: 40 mg Sodium Per Serving Range: 25-50 mg per 100 gm	High Sodium Range: 75-159 mg per 100
Asparagus	Artichokes, globe	Beet greens, cooked
Beans, green and wax	Dandelion greens, cooked	Celery
Broccoli	Kale, cooked	Chard, cooked
Brussels sprouts	Mustard greens, raw	Spinach, raw
Cabbage	Parsley	
Cauliflower	Spinach, cooked	
Chicory, bleached	Watercress	
Chinese cabbage		
Collards, cooked		
Cress, garden		
Cucumber		
Eggplant		
Endive		
Escarole		
Kohlrabi		
Lettuce		
Mushrooms, raw		
Mustard greens, cooked		

Exchange List
(no added salt)

List 2A: calories, protein, fat, and carbohydrate negligible.

List 2B: (per serving):
Calories 35
Protein 2
Fat 0
Carbohydrate 7

Okra
Peppers
Radishes
Squash, summer
Tomatoes
Turnip greens

Onions, mature
Peas, fresh, cooked
Peas, canned, salt-free
Pumpkin
Onions, green
Rutabagas
Squash, winter

Beets, cooked
Carrots
Turnips, white

Dandelion greens, raw
Peas, frozen, cooked

*Average: 5 mg Sodium
Per Exchange*

Starchy vegetables (per serving):
Calories 70
Protein 2
Fat 0
Carbohydrate 15

Corn
Parsnips
Potatoes
Sweet potatoes, fresh, cooked,
or canned, salt-free

included when calories are not restricted. The sodium content is approximately 2 mg sodium for a 1/2 cup serving.

Fruit juices are counted at 2 mg sodium per 1/2 serving. Unsweetened juices are included in the diet plan when calories are limited; sweetened juices when the calories are not limited.

Dried fruits, in the quantities listed as fruit exchanges in Section I, are included in restricted sodium diets at 2 mg sodium each. Dried apples, peaches, and pears, in quantities of 1/2 ounce each, may be included at the same sodium level. Dried apples, dates, peaches, pears, and prunes are at the low end of the range of sodium content. Dried apricots, figs, and raisins are at the high end and should be used less often.

Note: The calorie and carbohydrate values for fruit and fruit juices in the table of nutrient values for food groups used in restricted sodium diets are for unsweetened products as listed in the food exchange system. Sweetened products would be used only when calories and/or carbohydrate are not restricted. The sodium values average the same.

Pasteurized fruit and fruit juices may have sodium benzoate added as a preservative. State laws differ.

Bread-Cereal Group

Bread prepared without added salt contains some sodium, the amount depending on the kind and proportion of ingredients and on the local water supply. One product, developed in cooperation with a bakery in the Madison area averaged 5-1/2 mg sodium for a 1-ounce slice.

Breads prepared with salt vary widely in sodium content due to the above factors and the amount of salt in the formula. For example, one sample analyzed in the Chemistry Laboratories of the Wisconsin Center for Health Sciences contained over 200 mg sodium in a 23-gram slice.

If regular bread is included in the diet plan it is recommended that the sodium content of the local supply be determined either by calculation of the formula or by analysis. Mold retardants and other ingredients may contain sodium and should be included in calculated values.

Cereal exchanges include the following:

Ready-to-eat Cereals. One exchange at 2 mg sodium and 70 calories each.

| Puffed rice, puffed wheat | 1 cup |
| Shredded wheat | 3/4 biscuit |

Cereals to be Cooked. The quantities of cooked cereals and pastas (1/2 cup) listed as exchanges in Section One contain negligible amounts of sodium unless cooked with salt in water which contains an appreciable amount of the mineral. If one exchange (1/2 cup cooked) is included in the diet the sodium content need not be counted; the calorie, protein, fat, and carbohydrate values average the same as listed for the ready-to-eat cereals. The average weight, uncooked, of one exchange is 2/3 ounce or 20 grams. If larger amounts of the cereal or pasta are used as a serving (3/4 to 1 cup) under the above conditions the sodium content still need not be counted; but the calorie, protein, fat, and carbohydrate values would be 1-1/2 to 2 times as great.

Cereals and pastas included are: barley, corn grits, cornmeal (either white or yellow, whole ground or degermed), farina (regular or "instant-cooking"), oatmeal or rolled oats, wheat, rolled or whole meal, rice, macaroni, noodles, spaghetti. "Quick-cooking" farina and "instant" oatmeal are high in sodium. Read labels for current information.

Not included in a restricted sodium diet are all baked foods, either home-baked or commercially prepared, to which salt, baking powder and/or baking soda have been added.

Water. Softened water should not be used in food preparation. The usual method of softening water in the home replaces calcium with sodium. If the local water supply is high in sodium (more than 20 mg per quart) or if the diet is restricted to less than 500 mg sodium per day, distilled water should be used for drinking, for making beverages such as tea and coffee, and for cooking. If soft drinks are manufactured locally the sodium content of the product should be secured from the processor.

If distilled water is not used and if the sodium content of the water supply is over 20 mg per quart, values for the cooked cereals and pastas should be adjusted to include the additional amount of sodium. As a general guide, water is added at the rate of three times the measure of these foods.

Meat, Poultry, Fish

One ounce of lean cooked meat, poultry, or fish without added salt is one sodium exchange averaging 22 mg sodium. Kidney, brains, and sweetbreads are not included.

One ounce, weighed raw, of beef heart, calf, chicken, pig, or lamb liver, or one-half ounce of beef liver may be used as one sodium exchange.

Fish that is fresh, frozen or canned without added salt may be used; but frozen fish that has been dipped in brine in processing should be avoided. Labeling does not always indicate this possibility. If in doubt, rinse the fish in cold water. This will remove some of the salt.

Shellfish is omitted because of the high sodium content for most kinds.

Meats and fish that are smoked, salted, corned, pickled, or otherwise processed with added chemicals should be avoided.

Sausages, luncheon meats, dried beef, ham, and bacon are not included.

Eggs

One egg contains about 60 mg sodium. Three eggs a week are included in the low and moderate restricted sodium diets, and their value is averaged for the seven days. They may be used as such or in cooking.

Dried Beans and Peas, Nuts, Peanut Butter

Dry navy, kidney, and lima beans are comparatively low in sodium content. One-third cup, dry measure, of any of these may be used as a sodium exchange for the starchy vegetables.

Dry peas are higher in sodium and should not be used as an exchange. Most processed soy products have salt added.

Nuts are low in sodium content. Unsalted almonds, filberts, pecans, and walnuts range from a trace of sodium to 4 mg/100 gm. Unsalted peanuts are also low in sodium. Unsalted peanut butter may be used when calories permit, at approximately 100 calories and 3 mg sodium per tablespoon. Check the label.

Miscellaneous Foods

Cocoa (not Dutch process) and baking chocolate may be used. Candies made without salt, milk solids, or other sodium compounds may be used. Avoid products made with brown sugar, molasses, or corn syrup. Vinegar, unflavored gelatin, cornstarch, tapioca, contain negligible amounts of sodium. Herbs and spices may be used freely except those mixed with salt or monosodium glutamate.

Low Sodium Foods

Many low sodium products have been developed to meet the demand for ready foods. Read the labels for the sodium content of an average serving. Institutions should check the chemical composition occasionally. The following are some of the low sodium dietary products available:

Low sodium milk
Salt-free butter
Low sodium cheese
Fish canned without salt
Vegetables canned
  without salt
Low sodium peanut butter
Low sodium condiments

Low sodium bread, crackers,
  cereals, cookies
Dietary soups, no salt added
Low sodium salad dressings
Low sodium gelatin dessert
  powders and puddings
Sodium-free baking powders
Low sodium bouillon cubes
  and soup bases

Potassium chloride, the usual salt substitute for table salt (sodium chloride) is not a part of the sodium restricted diets.

Products That Contain Significant Amounts of Sodium

Some drugs contain sodium; many wines (particularly cooking wines) contain appreciable amounts, and some ingredients used in food preparation must be eliminated because of their high sodium content. A few of these are:

Sodium cyclamate; used as a non-caloric sweetener.
Sodium benzoate; allowed in some states as a food preservative.
Sodium bicarbonate; a leavening agent.
Sodium propionate; a mold inhibitor used in baking.
Sodium saccharin; a non-caloric sweetener.
Sodium sulfite; an anti-oxidant for commercially peeled potatoes.
Sodium hypochlorite; used in preparing hominy.

Sodium nitrite; used in some processed meats.

Monosodium glutamate; used to enhance the flavor of foods.

Baking powders that contain sodium bicarbonate (baking soda).

Foods to Avoid

Regular bouillon cubes and soup bases. Low sodium products are available. Commercially prepared soups, canned, frozen, dehydrated.

Cured meats, corned meats, smoked meats and fish, dried beef, luncheon meats, salt pork, salted sausages, commercially prepared baked entrées, TV dinners. Natural cheeses, processed cheese, and cheese spreads have high salt content. Cottage and cream cheese are lower.

Regular peanut butter. Low sodium peanut butter is available.

Salted peanuts or other nuts, pretzels, salted and flavored crackers, salted popcorn, potato chips, corn chips, hominy.

Olives, sauerkraut, pickled cucumbers, peppers, etc.

Condiments such as catsup, chili sauce, soy sauce, prepared mustard.

Convenience foods and prepared mixes of all kinds, unless low sodium.

Baked goods, either commercial or home-baked, that contain baking powder or baking soda. Yeast may be used as a leavening agent, and low sodium baking powders are available.

Sodium and Sodium Chloride in the Hospital General Diet

To accept the quantity of sodium as so much sodium chloride is misleading because foods inherently contain sodium in variable amounts. In addition, other sodium compounds as well as sodium chloride are added in commercial processing practice. See list of products that contain significant amounts of sodium in this section.

The amount of *sodium* taken daily by adults is given as 100 to 300 mEq (2,300 to 6,900 mg) by the National Academy of Sciences—National Research Council. This includes the sodium inherent in foods and that added in processing, cooking, and seasoning at the table.

Dahl (1958) recommends that anyone with a family history of hypertension ". . . adopt early in life a diet frankly low in salt." He said also ". . . tentatively I suggest that a maximum salt intake

TABLE VI-27

CALCULATED NUTRIENT ESTIMATES OF THE RESTRICTED SODIUM DIETS AS SERVED IN A HOSPITAL

Nutrients	Unit	500 mg Sodium Diet	1,000 mg Sodium Diet	1,000 mg Sodium 1,200 Calorie Diet	1,000 mg Sodium 125 gm Protein Diet	2,400-4,500 mg Sodium Diet
Food energy	Calories	2,170	2,155	1,195	2,570	2,310
Protein	gm	85	85	90	130	95
Fat	gm	75	75	40	115	95
Carbohydrate	gm	295	290	120	265	275
Calcium	gm	0.8	0.9	0.8	2.0	1.1
Phosphorus	gm	1.4	1.4	1.3	2.3	1.5
Iron	mg	15.0	15.0	12.0	14.0	14.0
Magnesium	mg	286	287	210	397	287
Sodium	mg	461	1,192	960	972	2,985
Sodium mEq		20	52	42	42	130
Potassium	mg	3,749	3,779	2,663	4,566	3,129
Potassium mEq		96	98	68	117	80
Vitamin A	IU	6,544	6,527	5,854	7,499	8,993
Vitamin E	mg	7.3	7.3	4.0	5.7	6.7
Ascorbic acid	mg	178.0	178.0	89.0	104.0	77.0
Folacin	—			Not calculated		
Niacin equivalent	mg	29.0	29.0	31.0	40.0	33.0
Riboflavin	mg	2.0	2.0	1.8	3.6	2.1
Thiamin	mg	1.6	1.6	1.2	1.7	1.7
Vitamin B_6	mg	1.9	1.9	1.7	2.3	1.9
Vitamin B_{12}	mcg	4.8	4.8	5.6	9.7	4.9

of 5 grams per day for an adult without a family history of hypertension might be allowed."

The menus for the hospital general diet that were used as a basis for calculated nutrient estimates have a three-day average of about 4,000 mg sodium (174 mEq). This includes approximately 3,200 mg sodium for the amount inherent in foods and the amount added as seasoning in food preparation and 775 mg sodium for two packets (1 gram each) of salt. These two packets represent an estimate of the amount of salt that might be used as additional seasoning by the person served. As a routine one packet (1 gram) was served with each tray except for diets restricted in sodium. See hospital general diet, Section Two.

The hospital meals as planned and prepared were moderate in respect to salt.

1. Foods, with the exception of breads, canned soups, a few salad dressings, and some accessory items, were prepared in the hospital production area.

2. Foods were lightly salted in preparation and some, such as eggs, not at all.

3. Seasoning of salad dressings made in the hospital production area was moderate in salt rather than extreme.

4. Herbs and spices were used as seasoning materials rather than condiments and sauces which may contain considerable salt. Monosodium glutamate was used only when included in soup bases.

5. Many foods that have a high salt content were not included in the menus. Cream, cottage, swiss, and cheddar cheeses were used. Snack foods such as flavored crackers, pickled items, and highly salted meats were not used.

Single analyses of water, brewed coffee, and steeped tea at University Hospitals in Madison were reported by Gormican (1970). The sodium values for 100 grams, respectively, were 3.8 mg, 0.86 mg, and 0.7 mg. When 1 cup (8 ounces) each of coffee and tea and 4 cups of water were added to the calculated nutrient estimate of the sodium in the general diet the total is this:

	Milligrams Sodium
Hospital general diet including salt on trays	4,000
Coffee, 1 cup	2
Tea, 1 cup	2
Water, 4 cups	36
Total for day	4,040

REFERENCES

SODIUM RESTRICTED DIETS

American Heart Association, Heart Disease Control Program of US Public Health Serv, and American Dietetic Association: *Sodium Restricted Diet, 500 milligrams, Revised,* and *Sodium Restricted Diet, Mild Restriction, Revised.* New York, Am Heart Assoc, 1969.

Cooper, GR; Heap, B.: Sodium ion in drinking water. 2: Importance, problems, and potential applications of sodium ion in restricted therapy. *J Am Diet Assoc, 50*:37, 1967.

Dahl, LK: Salt intake and salt need. *N Engl J Med, 258*:1152, 1205, 1958.

————: Salt and hypertension. *Am J Clin Nutr, 25*: 231, 1972.

Earley, LE; Daugherty, TM: Sodium metabolism. *N Engl J Med, 281*:72, 1969.

Lawton, GW; Busse, W: Drinking water, a source of sodium. *Wis Med J, 65*:259, 1966.

National Academy of Sciences-National Research Council: *Sodium-Restricted Diets: The Rationale, Complications, and Practical Aspects of Their Use.* Natl Res Council Publ 325, Washington, DC, 1954.

Newborg, B: Sodium-restricted diet. Sodium content of various wines and other alcoholic beverages. *Arch Intern Med, 123*:692, 1969.

San Francisco Heart Assoc, Inc: *Sodium in Medicinals. Tables of Sodium Values.* Prepared by Special Diet Committee, San Francisco Heart Association in cooperation with Univ of Calif Hospital Pharmacy, San Francisco Medical Center, 1966.

Schroeder, HA: Municipal drinking water and cardiovascular death rates. *JAMA, 195*:125, 1966.

Shapiro, S, et al: Fatal drug reactions among medical inpatients. *JAMA, 216*:467, 1971.

White, JM, et al: Sodium ion in drinking water. I: Properties, analysis, and occurrence. *J Am Diet Assoc, 50*:32, 1967.

Wilson, M: The influence of the diet prescription and the educational approach in patient adherence to sodium-restricted intake. *Med Times, 94*:1514, 1966.

DIETS IN DIAGNOSTIC PROCEDURES

ALLERGY: ELIMINATION DIET SEQUENCE

FOOD SENSITIVITY MAY BE DIFFICULT to diagnose because of the multiplicity of internal and external environmental conditions in which individuals live and breathe. Tolerances within the same individual vary due to the many combinations of factors present. If an allergic person experiences a lowered tolerance during the pollen season he may find it necessary to follow a more restricted diet at that time to maintain the load of allergens within the limit of his tolerance.

Diet histories have been found practical in assigning the cause of allergic response. Depending upon the severity of the reaction and the individual's recall of foods causing the reaction, a list is developed which omits all forms of the offending foods. These foods generally regarded as least likely to cause reactions are included in this list for trial. After the person is free of symptoms for a period, foods are gradually added, one at a time in graded amounts, until the offending food is identified. A diet record must be kept as directed by the physician. He sets the number of days for trial of the limited list of foods, and prescribes when new foods are added and what they should be.

Restricted diets should not be continued indefinitely without supervision. Supplementation, particularly of calcium, iron, and vitamins, should be considered.

Milk, eggs, seafood, wheat, orange juice, and nuts are frequent offenders. In families where there has been a history of food allergies, it is wise to delay introduction of these foods to the child's diet, then add in limited quantities till tolerance is determined.

220

Foods Less Likely to Cause Allergic Manifestations
(Rowe and Rowe, 1972)

Meat: Lamb

Fruit and Vegetables (All must be cooked except lettuce)

Apricots	Beets	Oyster plant
Cranberries	Carrots	Sweet potato
Peaches	Chard	
Pears	Lettuce	

Cereal and Cereal Products

Rice	Rice Krispies
Puffed rice	Rice biscuits (This is a special
Rice flakes	product available from Battle Creek
	Foods, Battle Creek, Michigan.)

Fats and Oils

Vegetable oil, including olive oil

Vegetable shortening (no margarine or shortening made from animal fat)

Beverage: Water (no tea or coffee)

Miscellaneous

Distilled vinegar	Tapioca
Salt	Synthetic vanilla extract
Cane or beet sugar	

No other foods or beverages may be taken. Chewing gum may not be used. No medication may be taken unless prescribed by the physician.

REFERENCES

Cole, D: Feeding allergic patients. *Hospitals,* 45:95, 1971.
Feingold, BF: *Introduction to Clinical Allergy.* Springfield, Thomas, 1973.
Fontana, VJ; Strauss, MB: Allergy and diet. In Goodhart, RS; Shils, ME (Eds.): *Modern Nutrition in Health and Disease.* Philadelphia, Lea and Febiger, 1973, Chap 33.
Rowe, AH; Rowe, A, Jr: *Food Allergy, Its Manifestations and Control, and the Elimination Diets—A Compendium.* Springfield, Thomas, 1972.
Waldman, TA, et al: Allergic gastroenterology: A cause of excessive gastrointestinal protein loss. *N Engl J Med, 276:*761, 1967.

200 MG CONSTANT CALCIUM DIET
FOR METABOLIC CALCIUM STUDIES

A constant and carefully measured calcium intake is necessary for several days prior to making calcium metabolic measurement as well as during the time that the study is being made. The dietary calcium intake must be constant for a period of two to ten days, depending upon the procedure used. It is essential that the constant calcium diet be continued throughout the entire period that measurements are made.

Any portion of the food not ingested must be measured and reported to the physician.

Only distilled water may be used for drinking, cooking, and preparing beverages. Foods are cooked without added salt, but 2 gm are provided for day's use.

The menu is identical for the entire period of the study.

Menu for Constant Calcium Diet

Foods	Amount	Calcium
Breakfast		mg
Grapefruit juice, canned, unsweetened	200 gm	16
Egg	1 large	27
Whole-wheat bread made with water	1 slice	21
Butter, 72 cuts to a pound	6 grams	1
Jelly, 1 serving packet commercial product	1 tablespoon	4
Sugar	As desired	0
Coffee, tea, decaffeinated beverage made with distilled water	As desired	0
Noon Meal		
Beef patty, broiled, no added salt	100 gm	12
Corn, canned or frozen, cooked without added salt	100 gm	3
Carrot sticks	20 gm	7
Whole-wheat bread made with water	1 slice	21
Butter, 72 cuts to a pound	1 pat, 6 gm	1
Jelly, 1 serving packet commercial product	1 tablespoon	4
Applesauce	100 gm	4
Sugar	As desired	0
Coffee, tea as above	As desired	0
Evening Meal		
Lean steak, broiled	100 gm	12
Baked potato	100 gm	9
Peas, frozen, cooked without added salt	100 gm	19
Lettuce	20 gm	4
with oil and distilled vinegar	As desired	0
Whole-wheat bread made with water	1 slice	21

Butter, 72 cuts to a pound	6 gm	1
Jelly, 1 serving packet commercial		
product	18 gm	4
Canned peaches, syrup pack	100 gm	4
Sugar	As desired	0
Coffee, tea as above	As desired	0
Total		195 mg
Two grams of table salt provided with breakfast tray to be		
used with the three meals		+5
Total		200 mg

Constant 100-gram Fat Diet for Chemical Fat Balance Test

The purpose of the test is to measure quantitatively the percent of ingested fat that is excreted in the stool during a period of constant fat intake.

The test period comprises 6 days; 3 days as a preparatory procedure and 3 days for collection of samples. The foods are the same for each day and include the following fat-containing foods in the amounts listed:

Food	Amount	Fat, grams
Whole milk	3 cups	30
Cooked meat	7 ounces	35
Butter, margarine	7 teaspoons	35
Total		100 grams

Other foods which do not contain fat may be served according to the person's desires:

Bread or dry toast, jelly
Fruit and fruit juices
Potatoes and other vegetables. Use fat from allowance only.
Gelatin desserts, no added fat-containing foods
Tea, coffee
Salt, pepper, sugar

Any portion of the fat-containing food not ingested should be measured and reported to the dietitian for suitable replacement. If the person is unable to eat, the physician should be notified. A daily calculation of the fat intake is made for the 6 days of the test period and recorded in the patient's chart. Interpretation: Normal individuals absorb about 95 percent or more of the ingested fat. In malabsorption syndromes such as chronic pancreatitis, postgastrectomy malabsorption, celiac disease, or non-tropical sprue, absorption is less efficient.

FAT-FREE SUPPER

A fat-free meal may be prescribed prior to a cholecystogram. This is usually served as supper preceding the morning of the test and may be one of the following menus:

Bouillon or other fat-free broth
Fruit plate with fat-free cottage cheese. This includes fresh (preferably) or canned fruit with lettuce and 3/4 to 1 cup fat-free cottage cheese. Mixing the cottage cheese with fruit or fruit juice will make it more palatable.
Toast or bread, and jelly
Angel cake without frosting, or fruit ice
Tea with lemon, black coffee, skim milk

*   *   *   *   *

Bouillon or other fat-free broth
2 slices toast and 2 servings of jelly
Fresh or canned fruit
Clear gelatin dessert or fruit ice
Skim milk, tea with lemon, black coffee

*   *   *   *   *

Dry cottage cheese on pineapple slice
Baked potato, no butter or other fat
Any vegetable without added fat
Toast or bread, and jelly
Angel cake without frosting
Skim milk, tea with lemon, black coffee

Sugar, salt and pepper may be on trays. There is no limitation on fluids. Not all of the food must be eaten. Quantity is not important. Omit all fat-containing foods such as meat, butter, margarine, salad dressings, gravy, whole or 2% milk, buttermilk, cream, peanut butter, ice cream, sherbet, non-dairy toppings, and cream alternates.

GLUCOSE TOLERANCE TEST DIET

Purpose: To test the ability of the body to absorb and metabolize glucose. A challenge load of glucose is administered orally, then at set intervals samples of blood and urine are obtained for glucose analysis.

Preparation of the patient:

1. The patient should be on a normal diet of about 300 gm carbohydrate for at least three days before the test.
2. He should be encouraged to have an adequate fluid intake to provide for an adequate urine flow.
3. He should have no food after the evening meal the night before the test. Water is permitted as desired but no other beverage.
4. The test is usually performed in the morning before any significant exercise.
5. The patient remains fasting throughout the test period except for controlled amounts of water (not more than 4 to 6 ounces per hour) to provide adequate urine flow.
6. He does not smoke or exercise during the test.

Performance of the test:

1. The patient is instructed to void and save the specimen. Immediately thereafter blood is drawn. This is the *fasting blood* specimen.
2. He is instructed to drink the entire glucose drink prepared for him. Time (hour) is recorded. The amount of glucose is as follows: Adults: Following laboratory instructions. Usually 100 gm glucose in 200 ml water (or equivalent amount of "glucola") Children: If less than 100 pounds, give 1.7 gm of glucose per kg of body weight in 200 ml water.
3. Blood and urine specimens are collected at the following intervals after the recorded time (in 2 above):

    30 minutes after ingestion of glucose
    1 hour after ingestion of glucose
    2 hours after ingestion of glucose
    3 hours after ingestion of glucose

    If reactive hypoglycemia is suspected blood specimens only are taken at 4 and 5 hours after the glucose is taken.
4. The blood and urine specimens are labeled and sent to the laboratory for GLUCOSE TOLERANCE TEST.

Interpretation: Fasting level of blood sugar is below 100 mg/100 ml
  Highest blood level is 160 mg/100 ml
  Time of highest value of sugar in the blood: 30 to 60 minutes
  At two hours it should be below 120 mg/100 ml.
Precautions: The patient may become nauseated or vomit during the
  test. If nausea occurs, it should be noted. If he vomits the test
  is terminated and the specimens are discarded.
Glucola: Simple solutions of glucose in water often cause nausea
  and delayed absorption. Commercial preparations, glucola
  and its equivalents which are tolerated better by patients, are
  available in pharmacies. Although these contain only 70 grams
  of glucose equivalent they result in essentially the same blood
  glucose response as 100 grams of glucose.

NON-PROTEIN BREAKFAST

FOR VITAMIN B$_{12}$ ABSORPTION TEST (SCHILLING TEST)

This meal is used as part of a procedure in testing vitamin B$_{12}$
absorption. It is served one hour after the administration of oral
vitamin B$_{12}$ and includes:

  Orange juice
  Toast with jelly (no butter)
  Beverage (no milk or cream)

One hour after the breakfast (2 hours after the oral vitamin B$_{12}$
dose) B$_{12}$ is administered intramuscularly. After this injection the
person may eat or drink as desired.

Results may be interpreted as follows:
  0 to 3% absorption indicates pernicious anemia or other cause
    of malabsorption.
  3 to 7% absorption is inconclusive.
  Greater than 7% absorption is considered normal.

DIET FOR TRYPTOPHAN METABOLIC STUDIES

Two types of tryptophan studies are sometimes done:
1. Studies on urinary levels of the serotonin metabolite, 5-
   hydroxyindoleacetic acid, used mainly for aid in diagnosing
   malignant carcinoid tumors.
2. Studies on urinary levels of kynurenine-niacin metabolites for

assessment of vitamin B₆ nutrition, estrogen-induced metabolic changes, or metabolic changes in patients with various diseases.

Dietary restrictions

Since both types of tryptophan study are frequently done together, diet restrictions for both tests should be the same. Omit the following items for at least 24 hours before starting the urine collections:

Bananas, dates, peanuts, peanut butter, liver
Soft drinks
Vitamin pills

Rationale

1. Hydroxyindoleacetic acid assay: Some, but not all, patients having malignant carcinoid tumors excrete elevated levels of 5-hydroxyindoleacetic acid (5-HIAA) as a result of increased serotonin synthesis by the tumor. Since bananas and dates contain interfering levels of these 5-hydroxyindoles, patients scheduled for this test must not receive bananas or dates during the urine collection period or for at least 24 hours preceding the collection.

2. Tryptophan-kynurenine loading studies: Tryptophan loading studies of the kynurenine-niacin pathway are usually done by collection of 24 hour urines before and after a 2.0 gram oral load of L-tryptophan (a normal and essential amino acid constituent of protein). Abnormal urinary levels of tryptophan metabolites are found in a variety of diseases, in pregnancy, in patients receiving estrogens or oral contraceptives, in vitamin B₆ deficiency, and perhaps in other conditions.

   The assay for metabolites of the kynurenine-niacin pathway are complex and may be subject to interference by sulfa drugs, phenacetin, acetophenetidine, and flavoring in many soft drinks. Since vitamin B₆ is involved in tryptophan metabolism to niacin, foods containing high levels of these vitamins (nuts, peanuts, peanut butter, liver in any form) must be avoided.

KEEPING CURRENT
WITH NUTRITIONAL LITERATURE

PRACTITIONERS DESIRING to be knowledgeable of recent advances in the field of nutrition can find no better resource than the *Journal of the American Dietetic Association*. Each issue carries original research and review papers. Approximately one hundred journals are reviewed monthly. Abstracts of articles pertaining to food, nutrition, food service management and related fields are presented. All of these articles are covered by subject and by author in each volume index. The section "Perspectives in Practice" describes advances of primary interest to the practitioner. The "ADA Reports," "Legislative Highlights" and "News Digest" note actions taken (and needs at the local level) in improving the quality of nutritional care, and, hopefully, in raising the sensitivity threshold of the beginning or isolated practitioner.

New books are reviewed in the *Journal of the American Dietetic Association*. Other recently released publications (including trade publications), films and training (learning) aids are described with information as to where each can be secured. All of these items are covered in the index listings of each volume, so these become one of the best, and certainly the most selective index to publications of interest to dietitians.

The advertisements are not covered in the volume indexes, but each issue carries an "Index to Advertisers". Careful reading of these advertisements (examples: nutrient content of oral and parenteral feedings, some with additional references; sources of special products for gluten-free, allergy, low sodium, ketogenic, and low phenylalanine diets; ready foods; labor-saving equipment) will give

228

the practitioner the armamentarium to speak knowledgeably to physicians and to others involved in management.

The *Annals of Internal Medicine* (Volume 79:393, 1973) has published "A library for internists: Recommended by the American College of Physicians." Although very short on many of the references regularly consulted by nutritionists, it includes a broad range of widely used medical journals and books in each area of medical specialty or sub-specialty. Each issue of the Annals carries a section on recently published "Literature of Medicine." The *New England Journal of Medicine* also covers a wide range of new medical literature in its sections on "Book Reviews" and "Books Received." Only the larger medical libraries catering to a broad range of medical needs will have a fairly complete stock of the literature cited.

The Joint Commission on Accreditation of Hospitals now requires that each *accredited* hospital have an easily accessible library with a range of references in the areas of service and a staff knowledgeable in how to secure desired references from larger regional libraries on inter-library loan. References needed by dietary services are being compiled.

Most hospital libraries will encourage use of their facilities by students and professional practitioners in the community, whether employed within the facility or not. College teachers are encouraged to familiarize their students with these specialized libraries to learn the type of assistance the medical reference librarian can provide. The institution's dietitian will welcome the opportunity to introduce students to the facility's library and librarian(s) and can assist in recommending publications related to the subjects desired. Such use of the hospital library will aid in familiarizing students with the hospital environment and personnel and may even help in promoting life-time patterns of library use.

Recent textbooks generally do an excellent job of citing the noteworthy literature up to approximately a year from the date of publication (adding to galley-proofs is costly). For example, *Modern Nutrition in Health and Disease: Dietotherapy,* 5th edition, by Goodhart and Shils (1973) is noteworthy for its selections of references from the medical literature.

Goodhart and Shils have written for students and practitioners in the fields of nutrition, medicine, and public health. The references abound with names of individuals from major research groups, individuals whom one can anticipate will publish advances as they take place, and will update their books to keep them current. The index cannot be expected to list every point desired (example: soy beans: nutritional value, research on, and implications for use cannot be found under these titles, but can be found elsewhere). With a good medical thesarus, a little imagination, and lots of perseverance, a wealth of knowledge can be gleaned on research related to clinical nutrition. It will be of great value to the specialist and the advanced student. Nutrition therapy for the infrequently encountered disease states which are not covered in less comprehensive publications can be found in this reference book.

Corinne Robinson's *Normal and Therapeutic Nutrition* (14th ed., 1972) is written for the student in the health care field and for the technically qualified practitioner, rather than the research specialist. It explains in easy to understand language the physiologic and biochemical concepts related to nutrition in disease. It answers the questions practitioners have as to the nature of the various disease processes and how to select foods to meet the needs presented. Food tables covering most of the newer vitamins and trace elements are included with citations to sources of data, and "additional references." A table on the amino acid composition of common foods is included.

In addition to selected references from nutrition and medical books and journals, Robinson's book also covers many of the nutrition related reports in the nursing literature, and government publications which are usually available in facilities with limited library resources and less emphasis on medical research. Nursing literature emphasizing the psychological and social aspects of patient care in the hospital, the home and the community is included. Nursing literature carries many articles valuable to understanding the pathophysiology of disease and deserves much wider use by nutritionists.

Many of the other texts mentioned among the nutrition references emphasize the biochemical aspects of nutrition, a foundation useful in clinical research and advanced academic work.

Keeping abreast of current nutrition literature can be accomplished in a minimum of time by:

1. Reading the abstracts in the *Journal of the American Dietetic Association* each month, and securing for study the desired original papers in the area of interest.
2. Using the standard indexes. For clinical nutrition the *Cumulated Index Medicus* (see particularly the section, "Bibliography of Medical Reviews") and the *Science Citation Index* cover a broad range of medical and nutrition literature. If literature in a specialized area is desired, the index of the journal of that specialty can be consulted. Many of these journals are included in the references of this book.
3. Consulting annual review serials. In this publication an effort has been made to cite annual review serials (*"Advances in ———," "Progress in ———," "Annual Review of ———,"* etc.) which might be of interest to nutritionists.

As the practitioner has already observed, clinical nutrition is changing rapidly. The development of the elemental (chemical) diet for oral use and of a synthetic formula introduced into a large vein for parenteral alimentation have brought about dramatic changes in the treatment of the patient with overwhelming disease or trauma. Likewise it has created some problems, which are being corrected, and has opened many avenues to needed research on basic nutrition and dietary interrelationships in nutritional care. For the patient with overwhelming disease or trauma, developments in tube feeding and the practice of using parenteral nutrition as an adjunct to the traditional oral feedings are hastening recovery and bringing a new era of hope.

Although the National Research Council "Recommended Dietary Allowances"—for healthy people—have been used for reference purposes throughout this text, it is recognized that few hospital patients fall into this category. A body of knowledge on effects of the disease process, and drug therapy is accumulating, but is not yet available for the many variables in clinical practice.

The lipid controversy is far from being resolved. Although there is general agreement on reducing calories, daily exercise and knowing genetic inheritance, there is not universal acceptance of some of the food selection (avoidance) advice being essential for everyone. Further epidemiological data and long term dietary studies will undoubtedly be forthcoming.

The spread between minimum levels of nutrients to prevent disease or poor performance, and the levels for optimum function and storage have been poorly defined. Recommended allowances in disease and trauma, and the effect of different nutrient relationships (including the effects of drugs on nutrient utilization) are gradually being developed. In fact this may be one of the major contributions of the next decade.

The traditional long-term use of the "bland" diet and the low residue or low fiber diet is well on the way to joining the archives of antiquity except for use in cases of open sores of the mouth or throat, and for patients to whom chewing and swallowing are difficult and painful. For long term use the palatable canned sterile liquid feeding of known nutrient content is frequently used in place of, or as an adjunct to, the full liquid diet or the so-called "smooth" (pureed) diet. In most gastro-intestinal disease, hydrophilic bulk rather than a low residue, or low fiber diet is desired. An elemental (synthetic) diet or a low residue diet of traditional foods is frequently used for a short period immediately preceding or following gastrointestinal surgery. Following hemorrhoid surgery the patient is more comfortable with a minimum of stool.

Dietary treatment in renal disease is also changing rapidly as dialysis becomes more available. Present practices vary widely from place to place, but undoubtedly will become more standardized, and probably less restricted, as experience with dialysis accumulates. The osteodystrophy often associated with renal disease has recently been found to respond to 1-25 dihydroxycholecalciferol (1-25 DHCC). Whether the osteoporosis of the aged will respond to this metabolite of vitamin D is being studied.

The impact of pharmaceutical agents on nutrition has scarcely been mentioned. Few generalizations are available, but as nutritionists become concerned with interrelationships, a body of knowledge is being developed. Bacterial composition for nutrients, the influence of various dietary products on gastro-intestinal flora, and the production of desirable nutrients as well as undesirable products are being considered. Drugs can interfere with metabolic processes in many different ways. It would be easy to think of (but hard to measure) competitive inhibition at metabolic sites, but who might have guessed that commonly used pharmaceutical agents might be the cause of flatulence? The selection of fruit juices to recommend following surgery is being studied. Time will undoubtedly clear up the conflicting report. See references following Section III, Liquid Diets.

Gas forming foods formerly were a subject of jest. The "gaseous foods" traditionally thought of as the dried beans, onion, and cabbage families were to be "avoided if they cause distress." This is easy to do when the offending food is in a recognizable form, omitted in the kitchen; difficult to avoid when widely used in staple ready food items. Perhaps the new (1973) labeling regulations, or changes in food processing, will remove the offending but as yet unidentified fraction. Food technology literature, not covered in this publication, will undoubtedly report these advances first. The "man in space" program has brought many advances in nutritional science and may speed discovery in this area.

Social changes affecting the traditional family life style, advances in food technology and high economic return on sale of snack foods, more disposable income, and vending have all had a tremendous impact on the diet and frequency of eating. The traditional "3 square" meal pattern is giving way to the 2 meals plus 2 snacks, or 2 meals plus 3 snacks in health care facilities. More frequently in free style living this becomes the "2 + 1" or "2 + 0" meal pattern or total "snacking!" Although it has not been covered in this publication, menus are needed to show how nutrient needs can be met with different eating patterns. Even nutritionists need to learn how to adapt food formulas to new food products, and menus to changing food prices as well as consumer preferences. Students need to learn how to use the food exchange system in developing formulas for such combined foods as pizza, and how to evaluate products by this method. Adequate labeling will make such evaluation shortcuts available.

One of the changes brought about by buying ready combined foods have been a marked increase in the salt content of the diet. Little original research has been published on the nutrient content of these foods as eaten. The toxicants in foods (such as nitro-samines) are receiving more attention in doctoral candidate research than the changes in nutrient content. There have been some reports of excess micronutrients caused by excesses in animal feeds.

The newer labeling regulations undoubtedly will give a tremendous volume of industry-financed data on food composition. A system of checking the reliability of analytical methods is needed. In due time a considerable volume of analytical data will be available for social and economic policy and planning action. Will nutrition objectives be a part of this action?

Appendix I — (Continued)

INFORMATION HELPFUL IN PLANNING DIETS
FOR INDIVIDUALS

FOOD PREFERENCES, CUSTOMS, AND PRACTICES vary widely among individuals and groups. Food products, and food and beverage availability continue to change. Social patterns are changing rapidly. As more food and beverage is consumed away from home it becomes imperative to identify the effect of these changes on the individual and to seek means to utilize all resources to promote good nutrition.

Nutrition education is valuable at any age, but to be most effective such programs should be directed to the family, the basic social group. Food habits are established early in life. Prevention or modification of conditions causing poor nutrition is the object of food education.

Although the genetic origins of disease are receiving increasing recognition, it is known that the sequence of untoward events can be materially slowed by good nutrition practices. For example, epidemiological studies have shown the need for many people to reduce caloric consumption and particularly to reduce total fat consumption.

In planning a nutrition program for an individual or for a group all members of the health team should take into consideration this background information:

1. The nutritional needs of each member of the family. Food plans should meet the needs of individuals requiring nutrients to cover the demands of growth, pregnancy, lactation, increased activity, disease conditions, malabsorption, and exceedingly high or low environmental temperature. They should also include the food needs of the individual requiring fewer calories to achieve and maintain optimum weight.

235

2. The family inheritance. If there is a familial history of high blood pressure, overweight, or diabetes, food habits should be promoted that will help to reduce controllable risk factors.

3. Conditions imposed by lifestyle: hours away from home, hours of work, demands of social situations.

4. The economic level of the family. Is money being spent wisely for good nutrition and the purchase of foods within the budget? Are the selection and purchase of foods being used for learning about food values in relation to cost?

5. The social needs of each member of the family.

6. Are children learning to accept a wide variety of foods? Are there opportunities for them to learn about food purchasing, preparation, and service?

Information to be considered by the counselor in food planning:

1. Consider all foods and beverages ingested in the day.

2. The eating pattern in relation to the day's schedule.

3. The distribution of the nutrients among the meals to spread food values and to avoid metabolic overload.

4. Promote moderation in the use of fats, refined sugars, *empty calorie* foods. Look for means to increase the use of fruits, vegetable, and whole grain cereals in the day's meals.

5. Recommend moderation in the use of salt and condiments and snacks high in salt. Suggest that the salt used generally be iodized.

6. Suggest restraint if caffeine-containing beverages are used.

7. Recommend a program of daily exercise.

PLANNING MENUS FOR HOSPITALS

The labor requirement of food preparation in a given institution is influenced by a number of factors:

1. *The planning of the menu.* The number of times included in a menu and the proportion requiring complicated preparation procedures are two affective decisions.

   The selective menu system may be constructed of two categories of choices:

   a. A basic general menu that is composed of plain foods simply prepared

   b. Alternate choices (mainly entrées, salads, desserts) that may be used to add variety and calories.

Thus there would be a sequence of plain foods with alternates of higher calorie value from which the person served may select according to appetite and liking. The plain foods in this selective menu can be adapted to the needs of a wide range of modified diets:

    a. Choices in either the basic general menu or the alternates may be of texture suitable for inclusion in the soft diet series.

    b. The plain foods are suitable for diets restricted in calories and may be used for planning diets in diabetes mellitus if portions are controlled in quantity, and concentrated carbohydrates are omitted.

    c. The combined foods may be used in diets at higher caloric levels.

    d. Provision of suitable low cholesterol, modified fat alternates for egg yolk, whole milk, cheese, butter, and fat meats will satisfy the requirements of diets qualitatively modified in fat and cholesterol.

All recipes should be standardized to a determined average portion and the nutrients calculated. Use of exchange quantities within the food groups in recipe formulation is of particular importance when using combined foods in a quantitative diet. When vegetables prepared for the general diet are seasoned with butter or margarine at the rate of 3 ounces per 100 servings, the quantity of fat per serving is less than 1 gram. Vegetables so prepared may be used for low fat or low calorie diets. Two to four servings of vegetables so prepared may be counted as providing one-half to one fat exchange.

2. *The degree of preparation of food purchase.* This ranges from raw material to ingredients partially prepared (kitchen ready) for further processing in the institution, to foods ready and portioned for service. It ranges from complete preparation to simple reheating of off-premise-prepared foods.

3. *The method of meal service*: Tray, table, or cafeteria, and the use of vending machines for ambulatory patients, for personnel and guests. This includes the proportion of single service (discardable) items used in the preparation and service of foods,

Table A-1—A Selective Menu Plan with Some Suggestions for Modified Diets

Foods in the basic General Diet Include foods useful for modified diets wherever possible	Alternate choices in planned general menu for patient selection	Alternates in same food groups for use in modified diets
Whole milk, skim milk	As requested	Low fat products for diets controlled in fat and/or calories; high fat for ketogenic diets
Cream, half & half, ice cream, whipped cream	As requested	
Cheese, cottage cheese, cream cheese, plain	In entrées, salads, salad dressings	
Soups, all kinds	As requested	Clear broth, pureed vegetable soups, soups with noodles, etc.
Lean meats, roasted, baked, broiled, simmered Fish, fresh, frozen, canned, in plain styles Eggs	Meat, poultry, and fish in stews, casseroles, salads, etc. Fried and deep-fat fried items. Sausages.	Plain meats, poultry, fish for diets controlled in nutrients; ground and pureed meats when required. Shellfish restricted in low cholesterol diets, eggs limited.
Potatoes, baked, boiled, mashed; vegetables with simple seasonings; fresh, frozen, dried, and canned fruit	Scalloped, creamed, breaded, fried, deep-fat fried items, potato chips;	Plain. Fats and seasonings within dietary allowances. Salads same as basic menu but limited in quantity for low calorie diets.
Salads of greens, raw or cooked vegetables, raw or canned fruit; raw vegetable sticks Vegetable and fruit juices, plain or gelled	Salads that are combinations of a variety of foods; jellied or frozen salads that are high in fat and sugar	Coarse-fibred foods, skins, seeds, omitted in soft diet series. Some soft textured and finely cut fruits and vegetables required.
Cereals, cooked or ready-to-eat, plain Pastas, rice, as alternates for potatoes Breads, rolls, biscuits, muffins	Pre-sweetened ready-to-eat cereals Also in soups, casseroles Sweet rolls, pancakes	Breads and cereals same as in basic menu but controlled in quantity. Some refined bread and cereals may be required. Sweetened products in high calorie diets
Butter, margarine, salad dressings	As requested	Controlled as to kind, ingredients and amounts.
Gravies, sauces	As requested	None unless fat free for fat or calorie controlled diets.

Sweets: sugar provided on trays jelly, jam, sweet sauces and syrup according to menu	As requested As requested	Seldom included if calories or concentrated carbohydrates are limited
Desserts: fruit either raw or processed; or custards, plain cake or cookies ice cream without sauce, sherbet, jello, angel or sponge cake.	As desired. Fruit crisps and puddings, iced or whipped cream cakes, ice cream with sauces, nuts Toppings, whipped cream or non-dairy	Unsweetened fruits for calorie or carbohydrate controlled diets. Limited portions of ice cream or plain dessert at higher calorie levels. No sauces or toppings for low sugar, low fat diets.
Salt, pepper, seasonings: salt and pepper provided on trays. Moderate salting of cooked foods. (See below) Moderate use of herbs, seasonings, spices.	Salt and pepper as requested. Occasional inclusion of a highly seasoned food such as barbecue sauce, chili, etc.	No nuts on some diets. Diets extremely limited in sodium require special selection and cooking without salt. A bland diet limits some seasonings and condiments.
Beverages: Coffee, tea, decaffeinated beverages	As requested	As prescribed
Condiments: Chili sauce, catsup, soy sauce, etc., according to foods on planned menu	As requested	As prescribed

Watt and Merrill (1963) list "moderate salting" of foods as 0.6 percent of the finished product. This is the amount usually present in canned vegetables.

and the number of articles included in a meal service. Examples are tray covers, saucers under cups, extra spoons and forks, cups or tumblers for milk, etc.

4. *Any duplication of an activity.* Individual on-site preparation of vegetables when a centralized service could provide measured quantities to cooking units is an illustration. Double handling of foods such as partial preparation one day, freezing, and reheating on a following day may spread the work to off-peak time, but may also increase the number of labor hours for the task. Elimination of steps is the goal.

5. *The degree of catering* to food preferences, and the number and variety of between-meal feedings. Requested variations from the planned menus can add work not only to the food service personnel but also to the purchasing and accounting departments. The number and kind of feedings throughout the day required by some therapeutic diets can require off-beat preparation and service. Multi-meal menu plans can decrease animal protein use and lower food cost by using smaller portions of the less expensive "extender" meat foods as alternates for the traditional noon or evening meat meal. This will influence mineral and vitamin intake. With a higher cereal diet, zinc, methionine and vitamin B_{12} must be watched.

Dietary Instruction

Selective menus are a tool for dietary instruction. They make the patient an active participant in his dietary planning. Selecting from a list of foods which may or may not be allowed in the diet prescription requires understanding of the principles of dietary prescription.

Communication between the patient and the dietitian concerning menu choices provides a more relaxed atmosphere. It focuses on an activity rather than an individual. By this daily process of selection common questions relative to the diet arise and are discussed before the patient leaves the hospital.

Table A-1 outlines a routine pattern for a basic general diet and gives some suggestions for alternates and a few changes for therapeutic modifications. Fundamentally, diets served in a hospital are divided as follows:

TABLE A-2

Nutritional Data*
on Oscar Mayer & Co Meat Products
Composition of 100 gm Edible Portion

	Calories	Protein gm	Total Fat gm	Fatty Acids		Carbo-hydrate gm	Cho-lesterol mg	Potassium mg	Sodium mg
				Satu-rated gm	Polyun-saturated gm				
All meat weiners	318	11.0	29.4	11.5	3.6	2.4	44	144	955
All meat bologna	317	11.1	29.3	12.1	2.4	2.2	38	138	900
Bacon (cooked)†	608	21.9	57.4	21.8	7.0	0.9	74	322	1900
Pork sausage (cooked)†‡	369	22.7	30.3	11.5	4.0	1.3	57	302	1367
Pure beef franks	317	11.1	29.3	13.0	1.1	2.2	48	130	891
Pure beef bologna	317	11.1	29.4	11.6	0.9	2.0	43	124	875
All meat cotta salami	233	14.6	18.5	7.3	2.0	2.1	41	172	943
Smokie links	304	12.8	27.0	10.4	3.0	2.5	42	161	838
Liver sausage (Saran®)	379	13.1	35.9	13.3	4.7	0.8	82	162	1045
Canned ham—Jubilee® (cooked)	129	21.1	4.8	1.7	0.4	0.4	29	324	1050

*From data presented in May and November, 1972. Courtesy of Donald Hoar, PhD, Nutrition Section, Oscar Mayer® and Co, Madison, Wisconsin. Further information on packing units, minerals, vitamins and fatty acids available from Oscar Mayer & Co.

Analysis was done by methods described by Eisner, J, et al: *J Assn Offic Anal Chem*, 45:337, 1962 and (Part II) Eisner, J; Firestone, D: *J Assn Offic Anal Chem*, 46:542, 1963.

†One lb as-purchased bacon will yield 0.31 lb cooked, ready-to-serve bacon. One slice of bacon cut 18 to 20 slices to lb will weigh 7 gm cooked.

‡One lb raw pork sausage will yield 0.44 lb cooked ready-to-serve sausage.

1. General diet. No limitation in kinds of foods, but planned to include the requirements of the daily food guide.
2. Modifications in consistency. Present liberalization of diets modified in consistency provides a wider selection than was possible in the past.
3. Modifications in nutrients: protein, fat, carbohydrate, electrolytes. Careful planning of the general diet can include a large number of items that may be used for dietary modifications. Differences in the mission of the institution and in the number and fields of interest of the staff will set the pattern of operation and influence the labor requirement. Dietary prescriptions which restrict amounts of protein (renal series) and kinds of protein (low phenylalanine), or electrolytes (low sodium or low potassium) will require original planning although some foods prepared for the general diet may be included.

FOODS, DRUGS, AND BODY PROCESSES

Krondl (1970) has pointed out that foods may affect the absorption of drugs and, conversely, drugs may affect the absorption and utilization of foods. Research in this field is active and further reports may be anticipated.

Investigation is being directed toward the effects of drugs and heavy metals on intermediary metabolism; to the loss of electrolytes in diuretic therapy (Laragh, 1970); to the effects of oral contraceptive agents; and to the effects of ethanol (ethyl alcohol) on enzyme systems, and protein and triglyceride synthesis (Lieber, 1967). Nitrosamines and sulfites are under investigation.

Feingold (1973) suggests that artificial flavors and colors may lead to hyperkinesis and other behavioral disturbances in children. He also links salicylates to allergic manifestations in some persons and lists foods which should be eliminated on a salicylate free diet.

MAO Inhibitors

Certain foodstuffs, especially aged cheeses, should not be eaten during treatment with monoamine oxidase (MAO) inhibitors which are used as antidepressant drugs. Aged cheese contains tyramine, an amine formed from the amino acid tyrosine by bacterial action during the ripening process. Tyramine stimulates the release of catecholamines, i.e., norepinephrine, epinephrine, and dopamine. These are normally oxidized by monoamine oxidase. With the monoamine oxidase inhibitor drug present this inactivation does not take place and a variety of life-threatening hypertensive symptoms may occur (Horwitz, et al, 1964).

In addition to aged cheese other foods implicated in a similar way are beer, wine, pickled herring, chicken livers, yeast, broad bean pods, and canned figs.

Levodopa (L-dopa)

Pyridoxine (B_6) interferes with levodopa used in the treatment of Parkinson's disease. The developer and manufacturer (Eaton Laboratories, 1970) advises that patients on levodopa should be warned to avoid foods that are high in vitamin B_6, particularly malted milk, mature beans and lentils, all bran preparations, wheat germ, oatmeal, bakers' yeast, sweet potatoes, beef liver, pork, tuna, bacon, and molasses. The B_6 enrichment level of cereals should be observed and any providing over 1 mg B_6 per ounce of dry weight avoided. Parkinsonian patients frequently consume large amounts of dried fruit to overcome constipation. To avoid excessive pyridoxine intake, patients should be warned to limit consumption of dried fruits.

REFERENCES

Butterworth, CE: Interaction of nutrients with oral contraceptives and other drugs. *J Am Diet Assoc, 62*:510, 1973.

Christakis, G; Miridjanian, A: Diets, drugs, and their interrelationship. *J Am Diet Assoc, 52*:21, 1968.

Cotzias, GC: Levodopa in treatment of Parkkinsonism. *JAMA, 218*:1903, 1971.

Eaton Laboratories: Clinical insights into Parkinson's disease. No 5, *Eating and Nutrition in Parkinson's Disease and Syndrome.* Norwich, NY, Eaton Laboratories, 1970.

Feingold, BF: Food additives and child development. *Hosp Pract,* Oct 1973, page 11.

Feingold, BF: *Introduction to Clinical Allergy.* Springfield, Thomas, 1973.

Horwitz, D, et al: Monoamine oxidase inhibitors, tyramine, and cheese. *JAMA, 188*:1108, 1964.

Israel, Y: Cellular effects of alcohol. *QJ Stud Alcohol, 31* (no 2): 293, 1970.

Krondl, A: Present understanding of the interaction of drugs and food during absorption. *Can Med Assoc J, 103*:360, 1970.

Laragh, J: Diuretics in the management of congestive heart failure. *Hosp Practice, 5* (no 11):43, 1970.

244   *Diet in Health and Disease*

Lieber, CS: Metabolic derangement induced by alcohol. *Annu Rev Med,* 18:35, 1967.
Marley, E; Blackwell, B: Interaction of monoamine oxidase inhibitors, amines, and foodstuffs. *Adv Pharmocol Chemother,* 8:185, 1970.
Mayer, J: Iatrogenic malnutrition. *Postgrad Med,* 49:247, Mar 1971.
————: Nutrition and Cancer 2. Problems caused by drugs. *Postgrad Med,* 50:57, Nov 1971.
Milne, AA: Food and drug interactions. *J Can Diet Assoc,* 34:40, Spring 1973.
Oral contraceptive agents and vitamins. *Nutr Rev,* 30:229, 1972.
Roe, DE: Drug induced deficiency of B vitamins. *NY State J of Med,* 71:2770, 1973.
Schmidt, AM: New regulations on vitamins and minerals. FDA Drug Bulletin, Dec 1973.
Van Woert, MH: Low pyridoxine diet in parkinsonism. *JAMA, 219*:1211, 1972.

Flatulence

Flatulence, causing discomfort, is a frequent medical problem. Carbon dioxide and hydrogen have been identified as major components of flatus with nitrogen, oxygen and methane as minor contributors (Murphy, 1964). Murphy identified dried legumes as the major offender, followed by cabbage and onions which are only about one-half as "flatulence producing" as dried legumes. *Immature* lima beans caused little flatulence. The manner of cooking did not influence the gas-producing qualities of the dried legumes, but raw cabbage produced more flatulence than cooked cabbage (Murphy, 1964). The quantity of the food ingested influenced the volume of gas produced.

Calloway and Murphy (1960) found that the volume of gas produced by different individuals following ingestion of cooked dried beans varied widely. Anxiety and stressful conditions increased flatus. Exercise which produced increased ventilation aided in the elimination of gas via the lungs, resulting in less flatus production. Respiratory efficiency of the subjects affected flatus, as did certain antibiotics.

Dry beans digesta appears to contain a component that in some manner interferes with the normal transport of carbon dioxide into the blood for clearance. This interference has been postulated as due to several mechanisms or combination of mechanisms: irritation of the gut wall, vascular constriction, foam formation, increased intestinal motility or inhibition of carbonic anhydrase enzyme (Murphy 1964).

Calloway and Murphy identified the flatulence-inducing fraction, as containing the characteristic oligo-saccharides, raffinose and stachyose. Humans do not have enzymes to break down these products, but a wide range of microorganisms do. Bacterial metabolism is thought by many to be the major source of intestinal gases. Rockland is studying Clostridium perfringins, "the principal intestinal anaerobe," as the primary source of gas and has demonstrated that raffinose and stachyose in dried legumes are not the primary stimulants (Rockland, 1968) as formerly thought.

Calloway and Murphy note that most of the gas forming foods contain sulfurous materials; the sulfide ion is known to inhibit action of the carbonic anhydrase enzyme. Further study on this factor, which may implicate a broad range of "hot" spices, is needed.

Because of increased need for legumes as meat additives and alternates, research on the flatulence factor proceeds at a quickened pace. Increased use of high quality legume products as meat alternates in the health care facility must depend on patient tolerance as well as economic considerations.

There is no categorical class of patients that cannot tolerate dried legume products. However, the above cited research would indicate caution in use for any immobilized seriously ill patient, particularly one suffering trauma, in respiratory distress, or one with disease of the gastro-intestinal tract. This research and other research stimulated by the "man in space" program is changing our concept regarding foods to present following surgery or other trauma (Hickey, Calloway, Murphy, 1972). With increasing lack of control over the food supply, it appears that the solution to identifying foods that are poorly tolerated is more complicated than the simple directive to "avoid the offending food." Until labeling is much more complete, it may be impossible to identify the "offending food." Some drugs, by prescription and by self-selection, influence the production of flatus.

REFERENCES

Calloway, DH; Murphy, EL: The use of expired air to measure intestinal gas formation. *Ann NY Acad Sci, 150* (Art 1):82, 1968.

Hickey, CA; Calloway, DH; Murphy, EL: Intestinal gas production following ingestion of fruits and fruit juices. *Am J Dig Dis, 17*:383, 1972.

Murphy, EL: *7th Research Conference on Dry Beans.* Held December 2-4, 1964 at Ithaca and Geneva, New York. ARS 74-32, Agriculture Research Service, USDA.

Murphy, EL; Calloway, DH: The effect of antibiotic drugs on the volume and composition of intestinal gas from beans. *Am J Dig Dis, 17*:639, 1972.

Rockland, LB: A search for a convenient assay method for the flatulence factor in dry beans. *Proc Ninth Dry Bean Research Conference,* Fort Collins, Colorado, August 1968. ARS 74-50, Agriculture Research Service, USDA.

Rockland, LB; Gardiner, BL; Pieczarka, D: Stimulation of gas production and growth of clostridium perfringens type A (No 367-6) by legumes. *J Food Sci, 34*:414, 1969.

BRIEF REVIEWS OF SOME NUTRIENTS ADDED TO RECOMMENDED DIETARY ALLOWANCES IN 1968 AND 1973

Magnesium

The magnesium in the human body serves in its structure and in metabolism. Of the 20 to 28 grams in the adult body about 60 percent is located in the hard tissues. Soft tissues account for 10 grams or less, and whole blood ranges normally from 3 to 5 mgs per 100 ml. This mineral is generally involved in cell activity and acts in relation to specific enzymes.

A deficiency of magnesium may occur if the intake is insufficient as in extremely limited dietaries or if there is excessive loss. Low levels of magnesium in the serum occur in certain clinical conditions including malabsorption. Diets that are adequate in other nutrients are usually adequate in magnesium. Legumes, especially soy beans, are an excellent source.

Magnesium in Foods

According to Manelo, Flora, and Jones (1967) the average American diet is estimated to contain about 120 mg magnesium per 1,000 Kcalories. The calculated estimates of calories and magnesium in the hospital general diets are as follows:

	Kcalories	Magnesium, milligrams
Adults	2,265	301
Pregnancy	2,641	409
Lactation	3,086	417
Infants 3 to 12 months	945	150
Toddlers 1 to 3 years	1,445	172
Children and young people	2,185	307

The utilization of magnesium is influenced by the form in which the mineral occurs in the food; by the presence of chemical substances in foods which may combine during cooking, mastication, or digestion to form insoluble compounds; and by the presence and amount of other food materials such as protein, fiber, and fat.

Water may be a source of magnesium. One analysis of the drinking water in Madison, Wisconsin, gave the value of 4.5 mg/100 gm (Gormican, 1970). At this level one 8-ounce cup of water provides 10.8 mg magnesium. Water, and beverages made with water, were not included in the calculations for nutrient estimates.

Table 5 in *Agriculture Handbook 8* (Watt and Merrill, 1963) was used for the calculated estimates of magnesium in the hospital diets. According to the authors, "The tentative values of the content of magnesium shown in Table 5 have been assembled to meet an anticipated growing demand for information on magnesium in foods".

Food processing alters magnesium values. If there is shrinkage as in the cooking of meats the unit value is higher for the cooked product than for the raw. If water is added as in the canning of fruit, the cooking of cereals, and the making of stews, jellies, and gelled products the magnesium content of the water should be added to that of the product for a total value. If the product is soaked in water, or cooked in water and drained, there may be some loss of magnesium.

Table salt is listed as having 119 mg magnesium in 100 gm. Commercially processed foods may have salt used in preparation or added as an ingredient. Table 2 in *Handbook 8* gives an average value for added salt in canned vegetables as 0.6 percent of the finished product. Frozen foods vary in magnesium content due to the methods of processing and to the amount of salt added as an ingredient.

The magnesium of salt added as an ingredient in cooking should be included in the total value; salt added at the table is a variable amount.

Average Values of Magnesium of Some Common Foods

Food Group	Amount	Magnesium, mg
Milk Group		
Whole milk	1 cup	32
Skim milk	1 cup	34
Cheese, domestic cheddar	1 ounce	13
Meat; Fish; Poultry, Eggs		
Cooked lean meats range in magnesium content from 18 to 29 mg in 100 gm with lean beef and lamb and beef liver at the low end of the scale, and pork (total edible, lean, roasted) at the high end.		
Lean beef, cooked	3 ounces	15
Chicken, white meat, stewed	3 ounces	16
Egg, large, 8 to a pound, raw	1	5 1/2
Values for fish and shellfish have a wider and, in general, a slightly higher range than the meats.		
Cod fillet, without skin and bones, raw	3 ounces	24
Salmon, pink, canned liquid and solids	3 ounces	26
Shrimp, cooked, boiled	3 ounces	43
Dry beans and Peas; Nuts; Peanut Butter		
Lentils................................ 80 mg/100 gm		
Dry lima beans................ 180 mg/100 gm		
Mature soybean seeds ..... 265 mg/100 gm		
Dry coconut .... 90 mg/100 gm		
Peanuts, roasted.............. 175 mg/100 gm		
Almonds........................... 270 mg/100 gm		
Peanut butter	2 Tbsp	55
Vegetables and Fruit		
This food group has the widest range: from 5 mg/100 gm for raw pared apple to 88 mg/100 gm for raw spinach.		
Crisphead lettuce	2 ounces	6
Carrot, raw	2 ounces	13
Green peas, canned solids	3 ounces	17
Peaches, canned syrup pack, solids and liquid	1/2 cup	7
Orange juice, fresh	1/2 cup	13
Potato, raw, not pared, 3/lb.	1 medium	51
Grain Foods: breads and cereals		
Whole-wheat bread	1 slice	20
Whole rye bread	1 slice	18
White bread (3 to 4% milk solids)	1 slice	5
Rolled oats, not cooked	1/4 cup	29
Rice, white, cooked	1/2 cup	8
Fats and Oils		
Butter	1 pound	9
Lard, oils, and shortenings not listed		

Food Group	Amount	Magnesium, mg
Sugar and Syrups		
Granulated sugar		Trace
Honey	2 Tbsp	1
Molasses, light	1 Tbsp	9
Molasses, medium	1 Tbsp	16

REFERENCES

Hathaway, ML: *Magnesium in Human Nutrition.* HERR 19, USDA, Washington, DC, 1962.

Nelson, GY; Gram, MR: Magnesium content of accessory foods. *J Am Diet Assoc, 38*:347, 1961.

Shils, ME: Magnesium. Chapter 6, Section B in Goodhart, RS; Shils, ME (Eds.): *Modern Nutrition in Health and Disease.* Philadelphia. Lea & Febiger, 1973.

Shroeder, HA; Nason, AP; Tipton, IH: Essential metals in man: Magnesium. *J Chronic Dis, 21*:815, 1969.

Wacker, WEC; Parisi, AF: Magnesium metabolism. *N Engl J Med, 278*: 658, 712, 772, 1968.

Zinc

Zinc deficiency results in stunted growth, abnormal growth of hair, decreased development of accessory sex glands, anorexia and poor taste sensitivity. Zinc is a component of many metal enzymes and metal proteins. As such it is essential for cellular oxidation and protein synthesis. A deficiency slows wound healing.

Zinc is thought to be related to the action of insulin and glucagon, and to the detoxification of ethanol; the exact mechanisms are unknown. Serum zinc concentrations are decreased in a variety of infections, malignancies, malabsorption syndromes and other metabolically challenging disease states (Li and Vallee, 1973).

Zinc is found in a variety of foods. Animal sources, particularly shellfish, meat and milk, are rich in zinc. Phytates interfere with absorption. Calcium can further decrease absorption by formation of a zinc-calcium-phytate complex. Other trace metals and vitamin B_{12} have an influence on its utilization.

REFERENCES

Fox, MRS: The status of zinc in human nutrition. *World Rev Nutr Diet, 12*:208, 1970.

Li, TK; Vallee, BL: The biochemical and nutritional role of trace elements. In Goodhart, RS; Shils, ME (Eds.): *Modern Nutrition in Health and Disease*. Philadelphia, Lea & Febiger, 1973. Chap 8.

Osis, D, et al: Dietary zinc in man. *Am J Clin Nutr, 25*:582, 1972.

Sanstead, HH: Zinc nutrition in the United States. *Am J Clin Nutr, 26*:1251, 1973.

Vitamin E

This fat-soluble vitamin is essential in the dietary of man as well as that of more than 20 vertebrate species. Eight naturally-occurring tocopherols have been isolated to date; and alpha-tocopherol can be prepared synthetically. All eight isomers show biological activity but in varying degrees in reference to the synthetic de-alpha-tocopherol acetate which has been assigned the value of one international unit per milligram.

A deficiency of this vitamin causes a variety of symptoms in the muscular, hematopoietic, vascular, and central nervous systems. The reproductive system is affected in certain animals but not in man. The normal resistance of red blood cells to rupture by oxidizing agents is reduced under conditions of vitamin E deficiency. In some children with kwashiorkor, megaloblastic anemia was found as well.

The amount of vitamin E absorbed is reduced if a condition interfering with fat absorption is present. This may be ingestion of mineral oil, biliary tract disease, pancreatic insufficiency, or malabsorption syndromes.

The need for vitamin E is increased when the intakes of fat and of polyunsaturated fatty acids are increased. Harris and Embree (1963) suggested the ratio of 0.6 milligrams alpha-tocopherol per gram of polyunsaturated fatty acid to protect against vitamin E deficiency in man.

Holman (1970) reaffirmed the earlier recommendation of Harris and Embree that the ratio of grams polyunsaturated fatty acids/ milligrams alpha-tocopherol be not less than 0.6. Linoleate content of adipose tissue changes on a high polyunsaturated fat diet. Witting (1972) points out that persons on a long continued high PUFA diet may have an increased vitamin E requirement for up to 4 years after the return to a normal diet.

It is suggested (Tappel, 1967) that adequate amounts of vitamin E in the diet slows the process of aging by protecting the body cells from the tissue catabolism which is associated with old age.

Selenium and certain antioxidants have the ability to function as a partial substitute for vitamin E.

Using the quantities of food available for consumption in the United States in 1960 Harris and Embree (1963) estimated the average daily intake of alpha-tocopherol to be 14.9 mg. The quantities of the foods in these studies were based on disappearance from the market.

Bunnel et al. (1965) calculated the alpha-tocopherol content of eight different representative menus in a range of typical calorie intakes. The intake of alpha-tocopherol according to these calculations ranged from 2.6 mg to 15.4 mg with an overall average of 7.4 mg.

The calculated estimates for alpha-tocopherol in the diets were based on values provided by Stanley Ames in a table prepared for publication in a chapter on vitamin E in Volume V of *The Vitamins* (Sebrell and Harris, 1972).Comparisons were made with the values listed by Martha Dicks (1965). Not all foods in the diets were listed in the table of alpha-tocopherol content used; and not all foods appeared in the form in which they were eaten. Appropriate substitutions were made if the food was not listed; and the food as listed was included in the calculations even if the preparation was not the same. The totals of alpha-tocopherol tabulated for the diets in this manual must be considered as rough estimates, and of use only to indicate approximate levels of this nutrient. *Nutrition Reviews* (Mar 1972) lists pitfalls in calculating vitamin E content of the diet.

Fats and oils differ markedly in their vitamin E value and fatty

	a-tocopherol mg in 100 gm	Linoleic acid (PUFA) gm in 100 gm	Ratio a-tocopherol, mg PUFA, gm
Animal fats			
Butter	1.9	2.6	0.73
Lard	1.7	10.0	0.17
Vegetable fats and oils			
Margarine, regular	11.6	22.1	0.52
Margarine, soft	—	30.0	—
Corn oil	18.7	53.0	0.35
Cottonseed oil	35.8	50.0	0.72
Peanut oil	15.6	29.0	0.54
Safflower oil	34.8	75.0	0.45

acid composition. Since the ratio between these two elements in the diet is of concern, especially when the polyunsaturated fats are increased, the ratio in each fat added should be considered. The following are the alpha-tocopherol (mg) to linoleic acid (gm) ratios as calculated from data by Ames (in Sebrell and Harris, 1972), Watt and Merrill (1963) and H & G Bul No 72 (1970).

The ratio of milligrams of alpha-tocopherol to grams of linoleic acid depends upon the total amount of each in the diet. The quantity of whole grain products and green leafy vegetables will greatly influence the total value of vitamin E. When these items are restricted and the polyunsaturates increased, the selection of a vegetable oil with a relatively high ratio becomes important.

Average Values of Vitamin E in Serving Portions of Some Common Foods

Food Group	Amount	a-tocopherol Milligrams
Milk Group		
Milk varies seasonally and according to the food of the cows.		
Whole milk, average value	1 cup	0.14
Skim milk	1 cup	0.01
Cheese	1 ounce	0.28
Meat; Fish; Poultry, Eggs		
Liver and salmon are good sources in the Meat Group; muscle meats, cod, haddock, and pike are less so.		
Beef, cooked	3 ounces	0.21
Chicken breast, broiled	3 ounces	0.31
Liver, broiled	3 ounces	0.54
Egg, 8 to a pound	1 large	0.55
Cod fillet	3 ounces	0.19
Salmon, broiled	3 ounces	1.15
Vegetables and Fruit		
In the average American diet vegetables and fruit provide about 11% of the estimated vitamin E value. Thin, dark-green leaves such as spinach and parsley rate high.		
Lettuce, leaf	2 ounces	0.29
Carrot	2 ounces	0.29
Spinach, raw, edible portion	2 ounces	1.43
Citrus juice, canned	1/2 cup	0.05
Potato, fresh, 3/lb.	1 medium	0.08
Bread-Cereal Group		
The nearer the food is to whole grain and the more of the germ contained the greater the vitamin E activity.		
Whole-wheat bread	1 slice	0.08
Enriched white bread	1 slice	0.002

Food Group	Amount	a-tocopherol Milligrams
Rolled oats, not cooked	1/4 cup	0.05
Rice, white, cooked	1/2 cup	0.19
Fats and Oils		
Wheat germ oil is an outstanding source of vitamin E; cottonseed, safflower, and sesame seed oil have high values, and corn, olive, peanut, and soybean oils have good values. Coconut oil is a poor source. Margarines have generally good values but vary depending on the kinds of oil used in the manufacture. The range given is from 3.3 to 15.8 mg in 100 grams.		
Wheat germ oil	1 Tbsp	22.79
Corn oil	1 Tbsp	2.62
Coconut oil	1 Tbsp	0.08
Butter	1 pound	8.62

Some of the tocopherol value of most foods is lost in food processing and storage, the more extensive the processing the greater the loss. Ordinary cooking, except deep-fat frying, does not reduce tocopherol content. Pasteurization of milk causes no loss; canning and freezing of foods do.

REFERENCES

Ames, SR: Isomers of L tocopherol acetate and their biological activity. *Lipids, 6*:281, 1971.

————: Vitamin E. Occurrence in foods. In Harris, RS; Sebrell, WH (Eds.): *The Vitamins,* Vol 5, 2nd ed. New York, Academic Press, 1972.

Bunnel, RH; Keating, J; Quaresimo, A; Parma, GK: Alpha-tocopherol content of foods. *Am J Clin Nutr, 17*:1, 1965.

Dicks, ML: *Vitamin E Content of Foods and Feeds for Human and Animal Consumption.* Univ of Wyoming Bul 435, Wyoming Univ Agri Exp Sta, 1965.

Green, J; Bunyan, J: Vitamin E and the biological antioxidant theory. *Nutr Abstr Rev, 39* (no 2):321, Apr 1969.

Harris, PL; Embree, ND: Quantitative considerations of the effect of polyunsaturated fatty acid content of the diet upon the requirements for vitamin E. *Am J Clin Nutr, 13*:385, 1963.

Nair, PB; Kayden, HJ (Eds.): International conference on vitamin E and its role in cellular metabolism. *Ann NY Acad Sci, 203*:1-247, 1972.

Slover, HT: Tocopherol in foods and fats. *Lipids, 6*:291, 1971.

Tappel, AL: Where old age begins. (A discussion of vitamin E in nutrition) *Nutrition Today, 2*:2, Dec 1967.

Witting, LA: Recommended dietary allowance for vitamin E. *Am J Clin Nutr, 25*:257, 1972.
Pitfalls in calculating vitamin E content of diets. *Nutr Rev, 30*:55, 1972.

Vitamin B₆—Pyridoxine

The term vitamin B_6 refers to a complex that includes three active and chemically different forms of the vitamin. The name *pyridoxine* was adopted in 1960 as the group name, and pyridoxal, pyridoxol, and pyridoxamine as the names of the three free forms of the complex. The publication (Orr, 1969) used in calculating the nutrient estimates of the diets and of the average values of serving portions of some common foods in this section lists the vitamin B_6 values of foods. From a practical standpoint there is little biological difference among these compounds since inter-conversion between them is active.

Vitamin B_6 functions in carbohydrate, fat, and protein metabolism although its major activities are most closely related to protein and to amino acid metabolism. A specific relationship exists between B_6 and the metabolism of tryptophan. It has been demonstrated that this vitamin is essential in over 30 enzymatic reactions.

The infant is born with a store of vitamin B_6. During the first month of lactation the mother's milk contains from 0.01 to 0.02 mg/liter; gradually this is increased to 0.1 mg/liter.

A marginal or low intake of vitamin B_6 may have a detrimental effect on the physical and mental growth and development of children.

One result of vitamin B_6 deficiency has been described as a partial depression of the immunologic response.

Certain medications such as penicillamine greatly increase the urinary excretion of B_6. Oral contraceptives may lead to a vitamin B_6 deficiency.

Absorption of B_6 is decreased in malabsorption syndromes, and pharmaceutical supplementation or increased quantities of pyridoxine from food sources may be necessary.

The calculated estimates of protein and B_6 in the hospital general diets are as follows:

	Protein, grams	B₆, milligrams
Adults	86	1.8
Pregnancy	120	2.2

	Protein, gm	B₆, mg
Lactation	134	2.3
Infants 3 to 12 months	45	0.8
Toddlers 1 to 3 years	60	1.2
Children and young people	105	1.8

Average Values of Vitamin B₆ in Some Common Foods

Food Group	Amount	Vitamin B₆, mg
Milk Group		
Whole milk	1 cup	0.098
Skim milk	1 cup	0.103
Cheese, domestic cheddar	1 ounce	0.023
Meat; Fish; Poultry, Eggs		
All values are for the raw product unless otherwise noted.		
Lean beef	3 ounces	0.369
Chicken, light meat	3 ounces	0.581
Egg, 8 to a pound	1 large	0.055
Cod, flesh only	3 ounces	0.191
Salmon, canned	3 ounces	0.255
Dry beans and Peas; Nuts; Peanut butter		
Lentils............0.600 mg/100 gm		
Dry lima beans ....0.580 mg/100 gm		
Soybean seeds ....0.810 mg/100 gm		
Coconut, fresh..............0.044 mg/100 gm		
Peanuts, roasted..............0.400 mg/100 gm		
Peanut butter	2 Tbsp	0.107
Almonds, shelled............0.100 mg/100 gm		
Vegetables and Fruit		
All values are for the raw product unless otherwise noted.		
Crisphead lettuce	2 ounces	0.031
Carrot	2 ounces	0.086
Green peas, canned	3 ounces	0.043
Peaches, canned, syrup pack	1/2 cup	0.023
Orange juice	1/2 cup	0.048
Potato, 3/lb.	1 medium	0.375
Grain Foods, Breads, Cereals		
The grain foods are not especially good sources but the frequency of their use makes their contribution important.		
Whole-wheat bread	1 slice	0.045
Whole rye bread	1 slice	0.040
White bread made with milk solids	1 slice	0.009
Oatmeal, uncooked, 20 grams	1/4 cup	0.028
Rice, white, uncooked, 42 grams	1/4 cup	0.078
Fats (oils are not listed)		
Butter	1 pound	0.014
Lard	1 pound	0.091
Syrups (sugars are not listed)		
Honey	2 Tbsp	0.008
Molasses	2 Tbsp	0.080

Vitamin B_{12}—Cyanocobalamin, Cobalamin

This water-soluble vitamin is essential for the normal functioning of all cells, and especially for those of the bone marrow, the nervous system, and the gastro-intestinal tract. It is involved in protein, fat, and carbohydrate metabolism, and particularly with the metabolism of nucleic and folic acids. A megaloblastic anemia may be associated with a vitamin B_{12} deficiency resulting from a disturbance in the metabolism of folic acid. A conditioned deficiency of vitamin B_{12}, owing to the lack of intrinsic factor in the gastric secretions, results in pernicious anemia. "The intrinsic factor appears to bind vitamin B_{12} and, with calcium, attaches the vitamin to the wall of the ileum through which it is absorbed" (NAS-NRC, 1968). Loss due to surgery of the factor-secreting portions of the stomach or in the absorbing surfaces of the ileum may bring about a deficiency.

A vitamin B_{12} deficiency may also occur in persons with malabsorption syndromes, with blind loops or with small bowel diverticula.

The average American diet appears to supply sufficient B_{12} to meet the recommended daily allowances, but people living exclusively on vegetables may develop certain symptoms as a result of low intakes of the vitamin, yet anemia is uncommon in this group.

Vitamin B_{12} in Foods

Vitamin B_{12} is provided chiefly by foods of animal origin, and occurs in minute amounts bound to protein. The vitamin is quite stable during cooking, but severe heating of meat and meat products may cause degradation. Soy products are low in vitamin B_{12} (and methionine).

The table (Orr, 1969) used in calculating the B_{12} estimates of the diets in this manual includes a wide variety of foods but not all in the form in which the food was served. Moreover, Orr advises that the values for this vitamin in foods are tentative. Therefore, the calculated estimates of B_{12} should be considered only as an effort to obtain a level of the vitamin in dietary practice.

Average Values of Vitamin B_{12} in Some Common Foods

Food Group	Amount	Vitamin B_{12}, mg
Milk Group		
Whole milk	1 cup	0.00098
Skim milk	1 cup	0.00098
Cheese, cheddar	1 ounce	0.00028

Food Group	Amount	Vitamin B₆, mg
Meat; Fish; Poultry, Eggs		
Beef, raw, lean, trimmed of visible fat	3 ounces	0.00153
Beef liver, raw	3 ounces	0.06800
Chicken, light meat	3 ounces	0.00038
Egg, 8 to a pound	1 large	0.00100
Cod, flesh only	3 ounces	0.00068
Salmon, canned	3 ounces	0.00586
Fats		
Butter		Trace
Lard		0

REFERENCES: Vitamins B_6 and B_{12}

Brown, RR: Normal and pathological conditions which may alter human requirements for vitamin B_6. *J Agric Food Chem, 20*:498, 1972.

Harding, MG; Crooks, H: Lesser known vitamins in foods. *J Am Diet Assoc, 38*:240, 1961.

Lichtenstein, H; Beloian, A; Murphy, EW: *Vitamin B_{12} Microbiological Assay Methods and Distribution in Selected Foods.* HERR No 113, Washington, DC, USDA Agri Res Serv, 1961.

Meyer, BH; Mysinger, MA; Wodarsky, LA: Pantothenic acid and B_6 in beef. *J Am Diet Assoc, 54*:122, 1969.

Orr, ML: *Pantothenic Acid, Vitamin B_6 and Vitamin B_{12} in Foods.* HERR No 36, Washington DC, USDA Agri Res Serv, 1969.

Polansky, MM: Vitamin B_6 component in fresh and dried vegetables. *J Am Diet Assoc, 54*:118, 1969

Folacin—Folic Acid, Pteroylmonoglutamic Acid

This water-soluble vitamin is required for growth, reproduction, and the prevention of anemia in animals and of several types of anemia in man. Vitamin B_{12} appears involved in certain of the reactions in which folacin serves as a coenzyme.

A deficiency of folacin results in megaloblastic anemia, glossitis, and diarrhea; and a folacin deficiency may be due to inadequate dietary intake, impaired absorption, excessive demands by tissues of the body, and metabolic derangements. A high percentage of patients with malabsorption syndromes have impaired absorption of folacin. In tropical sprue, combined folacin and vitamin B_{12} deficiencies often occur.

The absorption of dietary folate possibly varies from time to time even in the same person because of changes in the intestinal conjugase concentration, intestinal pH, or the presence of inhibitor substances in the diet (cellulose, for example) which may have a selective affinity for various folate conjugates.

The requirement for folacin is increased in pregnancy, in various disease states, and by the consumption of alcohol.

Folacin in Foods

Determinations of folacin in foods have been made by bacterial assay; L. casei and S. faecalis have been used (Toepfer, et al, 1951). This publication shows a wide range of values not only from food to food but also among different samples of the same kind of food. Since this book was written there have been changes in the methods used for the assay of the vitamin. Hurdle, Barton, and Searles (1968) include a table comparing some published values of a number of uncooked foods. In this table the foods assayed by the more recent methods show the higher values.

Losses in folates may occur as a result of cooking, for some are unstable when heated. Hurdle, et al list the folate content of a number of foods in fresh or cooked states as served in a hospital dietary, and include a table showing the values of certain foods in the fresh state and when cooked by household methods. Neither boiling nor frying caused any loss in lamb liver or white of egg, nor did frying in white meat of chicken. Pasteurized milk showed no loss when just brought to the boiling point. There were considerable losses in cooked potato, cabbage, broccoli, oatmeal, and egg yolk.

Toepfer, et al summarizes the folic acid content of foods as follows: One milligram or more of folic acid in 100 grams of food, *dry weight*

Brewer's yeast	Asparagus	Leaf lettuce
Liver concentrate	Broadleaf endive	Spinach
Chicken liver	Calabrese broccoli	

From 0.4 to 1.0 mg folic acid in 100 grams of food, *dry weight*

Liver	Dry beans
Blackeye peas	Soy flour
Most of the other leafy greens.	

From 0.1 to 0.4 mg folic acid in 100 grams of food, *dry weight*
A few fruits and other vegetables except root vegetables.
   Thirty-five items in this group.

From 0.03 to 0.1 mg folic acid in 100 grams of food, *dry weight*

Root vegetables	Nuts

Most fresh fruits   Lean beef
Grains and grain products
Foods with 0.03 mg folic acid or less in 100 grams, *dry weight*
Eggs   Meat (other than beef)
Milk   Poultry

REFERENCES

Butterfield, S; Calloway, DH: Folacin in wheat and selected foods, *J Am Diet Assoc 60*:310, 1972.

Butterworth, CE, Jr: The availability of food folate. *Brit J Haematol, 14*: 339, 1969.

Hoppner, K; Lampi, B; Perrin, DE: Folacin activity of frozen convenience foods. *J Am Diet Assoc, 63*:537,1973.

Hurdle, AD; Barton, D; Searles, IH: A method for measuring folate in foods and its application to a hospital diet. *Am J Clin Nutr, 21*:1202, 1968.

Retief, FP: Urinary folate excretion after ingestion of Pteroylmonoglutamic acid and food folate. *Am J Clin Nutr, 22*:3, 352, 1969.

Santini, R; Brewster, C; Butterworth, CE, Jr: The distribution of folic acid active compounds in individual foods. *Am J Clin Nutr, 14*:205, 1964.

Streiff, RR: Folate levels in citrus and other juices. *Am J Clin Nutr, 24*: 1390, 1971.

Toepfer, EW; Zook, EG; Orr, ML; Richardson, LR: *Folic Acid Content of Foods*. USDA Handbook 29, Washington, DC, 1951.

NOTE: Robinson, CH: *Normal and Therapeutic Nutrition,* 14th ed. New York, Macmillan, 1972 includes food composition tables for most of the nutrients in the Recommended Dietary Allowances.

METHOD USED FOR ESTIMATING
NUTRIENT VALUES IN HOSPITAL DIETS

THE OBJECTIVES IN MAKING these calculations were to estimate the nutrient levels of diets as served in the hospital, and to provide information for revision of the dietary patterns or for supplementation if needed. The estimates listed are averages calculated from the foods planned for three days (Tuesday, Wednesday, Thursday) of one cycle menu in use during 1968 at the University of Wisconsin Medical Center (now Wisconsin Center for Health Sciences). They represent a dietary pattern in kind and amount of food and are subject to variations depending on a patient's choice of foods, on requests for smaller or larger portions, and on dietary prescriptions.

The quantities of foods used as bases for the calculations are as follows:

1. Standard units such as a slice of bread (1/20 of a pound), a pat of butter (72 cuts to a pound), one-half pint of milk, serving packets of sugar (4-1/4 gm), salt (1 gm), jelly, certain salad dressings, oranges of specific size.
2. Standard portions of meat, poultry, fish based on the dietary pattern of three ounces cooked weight at dinner, and two ounces cooked weight at lunch or supper. Meats are trimmed to "separable lean" condition.
3. Standard portions of processed fruits and vegetables: 12 servings to a 46-ounce can of juice; 5 servings to a pound of a frozen vegetable; 3 ounces of drained solids of a canned vegetable like peas, 4 ounces of solids and liquids of products like canned tomatoes.
4. Eight servings to a quart of cooked cereal of standard proportion.
5. Ice cream and sherbet in cups packed by the University of Wisconsin Dept. of Food Science and Industries. The cups are 3 fluid ounces in size; the ice cream averages 55 grams a portion, the sherbet 75 grams.

6. Average portions of foods prepared in the Production Unit from standardized recipes for soups, entrées, salads, desserts and other combined foods.

Random weighings were done on the portions of foods served for the daily sample trays and compared with the listed standard portions. Weights for solid foods were calculated in grams in most cases, in ounces for a few. Measures for liquids were converted to gram weights. Calculations were rounded to the same number of places as in the table of food values used.

The calculated nutrient estimates of the diets in this manual are listed for reference with appropriate recommended dietary allowances (See Table of Contents). This listing does not intend that the use of a diet should be limited to the age level shown with it. The purpose is to provide a relationship between the recommended dietary allowances and the diet plans. This correlation is summarized as follows:

Hospital menus used as bases for calculated nutrient estimates.	*Age levels of recommended dietary allowances listed with estimates.*
Diet for infants 3 to 12 months	Infants from 2 to 6 months
Diet for toddlers 1 to 3 years	Children 1 to 3 years
Diet for children and youth	Children 7 to 10 years
General diet for adults	Man 23 to 50 years, woman 23 to 50 years
Diets during pregnancy or lactation	Woman 23+ years
Modifications of the general diet	Man 23 to 50 years, woman 23 to 50 years

The energy values of the calculated nutrient estimates are based on those listed for specific foods in Table 1, *Handbook No 8.* Table No. 6 in the same publication shows the factors used in calculating the energy values for specific foods and for groups of foods. The sum of multiplications of the listed protein, fat, and carbohydrate values by 4, 9, and 4 (the rounded caloric values for protein, fat, and carbohydrate in common use) do not coincide in most cases with the listed energy value. Similarly, calculations of the protein, fat, and carbohydrate values of the nutrient estimates and of the diet plans by 4, 9, and 4 respectively do not agree with the listed energy value. For example, the factor to be applied for ingested cane or beet sugar is 3.85 calories per gram.

Comments on Tables of Food Composition

It is understood that there are many variables in the nutrient values of foods as eaten. The biological variation of the foods them-

selves may range within wide limits (Ohlson, 1972); and the day-
by-day changes in food preparation and service may result in
alterations in concentration and amounts of average portions. Moreover, since hospital diets are adapted to meet individual needs and
desires, some of these changes may cause marked variations from
the calculated nutrient estimates.

Estimates of the amounts of nutrients present in food materials
depend on tables of food values, and these depend on the method
of assay and on the samples included in the listed average. In some
cases the value for one sample only may be given; in others there
may be many samples included in the average. Individual samples
from different parts of the nation may vary. Age, condition, and
length of time of storage influence results. Processing methods of
foods differ. Formulas of prepared ready-to-eat foods vary not only
from processor to processor but also from time to time by the same
processor. Standards set by the U.S. Dept. of Agriculture for certain
food materials, i.e., mayonnaise, certain canned fruits and vegetables, assure reasonable similarity of major ingredients but changes
in processing methods and equipment used, and choice among
optional ingredients may alter in some way the nutrient value of
the product.

In addition, tables of food values, especially those that list the
values of the nutrients recently included in the recommended dietary
allowances, may not show all the foods included in a diet, or may
not show the value of the food in the form in which it was eaten.
An attempt has been made to use the tables to the best advantage.

REFERENCE

Ohlson, MA: *Handbook of Experimental and Therapeutic Diets,* 2nd ed.
Minneapolis, Burgess, 1972.

APPENDIX III

MEASURES AND WEIGHTS

Household measures and weights

Weights of these measures will vary with the density of the product. The following are approximately correct for water or milk.

1 tablespoon	3 teaspoons
	1/2 ounce
1 cup	48 teaspoons
	16 tablespoons
	8 ounces
1 pint	2 cups
	16 ounces
	1 pound
1 quart	4 cups
	2 pints

Approximate equivalents

1 ounce	30 grams
1 teaspoon	5 grams
1 tablespoon	15 grams
1 cup	240 grams

Metric measures and weights

1 microgram (mcg)	1/1,000,000 gram
1 milligram (mg)	1/1000 gram
1 gram (gm)	1/1000 kilogram
1 milliliter (ml)	1/1000 liter
1 millimeter (mm)	1/1000 meter
1 centimeter (cm)	1/100 meter
1 kilogram (kg)	2.2 pounds
1 centimeter (cm)	0.4 inch
1 meter (m)	39.37 inches

In practical use 1 milliliter is considered equal to 1 cubic centimeter (cc), and 1 cc is counted as 1 gram.

1 liter (1)	0.908 dry quart
* * * * *	1.06 liquid quart
1 ounce (oz)	28.35 gm
1 pound (lb)	453.59 gm
1 quart (qt)	0.946 liter

Measures of Energy

A kilocalorie (Kcal, or the large calorie) is the unit used in expressing the energy-producing value of foods. This is the amount of heat necessary to raise the temperature of 1 kg of water from 15° to 16° centigrade. One gram of protein = 4 Kcal; 1 gram of fat = 9 Kcal; 1 gram of carbohydrate = 4 Kcal.

The small calorie is the amount of heat required to raise the temperature of 1 gram of water 1° centigrade at a pressure of 1 atmosphere. One kilocalorie equals 1,000 small calories.

A joule (J) is a unit of work or energy approximately equal to 0.24 small calorie or 0.738 foot-pound. A foot-pound is a unit of work or energy equal to the work of raising one pound avoirdupois the height of one foot against the force of gravity. One calorie equals 4.18 joules.

263

CONVERSION FACTORS

Vitamin A

One international unit of vitamin A is 0.344 mcg of pure vitamin A acetate, or 0.6000 mcg pure beta carotene. These values were established in the rat.

Recent emphasis has been on expressing vitamin A values in terms of retinol equivalents. Rodriguez and Irwin (1972) use the value of 1 IU of vitamin A as equivalent to 0.3 micrograms retinol, and 1 microgram all-trans B-carotene as equivalent to 0.167 micrograms all-trans retinol. However, they point out that other mixed carotenoids with vitamin A activity are equivalent to .0835 micrograms all-trans retinol. Until there is sufficient information on the retinol equivalent value of foods, the NRC-NAS standard in IU will be used for general diets. It allows for a large proportion of the allowance to be covered by carotene from vegetable sources.

An FAO/WHO Technical Report (1967) reviews factors in the consumption pattern which influences the availability and utilization of vitamin A in foods. Little data are available on the influence of stress or disease on utilization.

Vitamin D

The USP unit of vitamin D and the international unit of vitamin D are identical. One IU of vitamin D is 0.025 mcg of pure vitamin D_3.

Niacin

Niacin values are given in the table of recommended dietary allowances in terms of milligram equivalents. One niacin equivalent is defined as 1 milligram of niacin or 60 milligrams of dietary tryptophan. Proteins of animal origin (milk, eggs, meat) contain approximately 1.4 percent of tryptophan, and proteins of vegetable origin (cereals, legumes) contain about 1 percent of tryptophan. In practical use one percent of the protein of an average mixed diet is calculated as tryptophan. This value, divided by 60, is added to the preformed niacin in the diet for total niacin equivalents.

Temperature

To convert degrees Fahrenheit to degrees centigrade, subtract 32 and multiply by 5/9. To convert degrees centigrade to degrees Fahrenheit, multiply by 9/5 and add 32.

MEASURES OF ELECTROLYTES IN FOODS

A mol (M) of a substance is the molecular weight of that substance in grams. One millimol (mM) is 1/1000 of this weight.

An equivalent of an ion is its atomic weight divided by its valence. One milliequivalent (mEq) is 1/1000 of an equivalent. For the univalent ion this is the same as the millimol. For the divalent ion the atomic weight must be divided by 2 to give the equivalent. One-thousandth (1/1000) of this value equals one milliequivalent.

Electrolytes in foods may be expressed as milliequivalents. This is the measure of the combining power, or weight, of the ion; and the milliequivalents in foods and dietaries can be compared with milliequivalent values of similar ions in blood and urine. The equivalent weight (Eq) is the atomic weight divided by the valence.

To convert milligram weights of sodium, potassium, and other monovalent ions in foods to corresponding milliequivalents, divide the weight of the element in milligrams by the equivalent weight of the ion—i.e., the atomic weight.

To convert milligram weights or divalent ions such as calcium and magnesium in foods divide the atomic weight by 2, and then

Ion	Atomic Weight	Valence	Weight in mg of ion in general diet	Equivalent Weight	Milliequivalents of ion in general diet
Sodium	23	1	3,952	23	172
Potassium	39	1	2,995	39	77
Calcium	40	2	1,100	20	55
Magnesium	24.3	2	301	12.2	25
Phosphorus	31	1.8	1,460	17.2	84.8

Phosphorus exists in the blood as both monovalent ion (H_2Po_4) and bivalent phosphate ion (HPo_4). At normal blood pH of 7.4, the average valence is 1.8.

One osmol (or osmole, Osm): one mol x number of ions formed by dissociation. Example: 58.5 gms Nacl equals one mol, but two osmols since Nacl dissociates into Na+ (23 gm) and cl— (35.5 gm).

One milliosmol (mOsm) 1/1000 osmol.

A mol*al* solution contains one mol of solute per 1000 gm of solvent. Since it is based on weight, not volume, the ratio of solute to solvent remains constant.

An osmo*lar* solution contains one mol solute to which a solvent is added *to make one liter of solution.*

Thus osmolality is the osmotic pressure in terms of osmols or milliosmols of solute per kilogram of solvent.

Osmolarity is osmotic pressure in terms of osmols or milliosmols of solute *per liter of solution.*

divide the milligram weight of the food by that value. In the following examples the weights of the elements in a representative diet are used as a basis for the calculations.

CONVERSION TABLE
SODIUM—POTASSIUM—PHOSPHORUS

Milligrams to milliequivalents

Milligrams	Sodium mEq	Potassium mEq	Phosphorus mEq
1	.043	.025	.058
2	.087	.051	.116
3	.130	.077	.175
4	.174	.103	.232
5	.217	.128	.291
6	.261	.152	.349
7	.304	.179	.407
8	.348	.205	.465
9	.391	.231	.524
10	.435	.256	.581
11	.478	.282	.639
12	.522	.308	.697
13	.565	.333	.755
14	.609	.359	.813
15	.652	.384	.872
16	.696	.410	.930
17	.739	.436	.988
18	.782	.461	1.05
19	.826	.487	1.10
20	.869	.513	1.16
21	.913	.539	1.22
22	.967	.564	1.28
23	1.00	.590	1.34
24	1.04	.615	1.39
25	1.09	.641	1.45
100	4.35	2.54	5.81
200	8.70	5.13	11.62
300	13.04	7.69	17.44

REFERENCES

Ames, SR; Harper, AE: The joule, unit of energy. *J Am Diet Assoc, 57*: 415, 1970.

FAO/WHO: Requirements of vitamin A, thiamine, riboflavin, and niacin. FOA Nutrition Meet Report Series no 41, WHO Tech Report Series no 362, Geneva, Switzerland, 1967.

Hoffman, WS: *The Biochemistry of Clinical Medicine*, 4th ed. Chicago, Year Book Medical Publishers, 1970.

Rodriguez, MS; Irwin, MI: A conspectus of research on vitamin A requirements of man. *J Nutr, 102*:909, 1972.

Vawter, SM; DeForest, RE: The international metric system and medicine. *JAMA, 218*:723, 1971.

DESIRABLE WEIGHTS FOR ADULTS*

Weight in Pounds According to Frame (In Indoor Clothing)

	HEIGHT (with shoes on) 1-inch heels		SMALL FRAME	MEDIUM FRAME	LARGE FRAME
	Feet	Inches			
Men	5	2	112-120	118-129	126-141
of Ages 25	5	3	115-123	121-133	129-144
and Over	5	4	118-126	124-136	132-148
	5	5	121-129	127-139	135-152
	5	6	124-133	130-143	138-156
	5	7	128-137	134-147	142-161
	5	8	132-141	138-152	147-166
	5	9	136-145	142-156	151-170
	5	10	140-150	146-160	155-174
	5	11	144-154	150-165	159-179
	6	0	148-158	154-170	164-184
	6	1	152-162	158-175	168-189
	6	2	156-167	162-180	173-194
	6	3	160-171	167-185	178-199
	6	4	164-175	172-190	182-204

	HEIGHT (with shoes on) 2-inch heels		SMALL FRAME	MEDIUM FRAME	LARGE FRAME
	Feet	Inches			
Women	4	10	92- 98	96-107	104-119
of Ages 25	4	11	94-101	98-110	106-122
and Over	5	0	96-104	101-113	109-125
	5	1	99-107	104-116	112-128
	5	2	102-110	107-119	115-131
	5	3	105-113	110-122	118-134
	5	4	108-116	113-126	121-138
	5	5	111-119	116-130	125-142
	5	6	114-123	120-135	129-146
	5	7	118-127	124-139	133-150
	5	8	122-131	128-143	137-154
	5	9	126-135	132-147	141-158
	5	10	130-140	136-151	145-163
	5	11	134-144	140-155	149-168
	6	0	138-148	144-159	153-173

For girls between 18 and 25, subtract 1 pound for each year under 25.

*Courtesy of the Metropolitan Life Insurance Company. In *Four Steps to Weight Control.* New York, Metropolitan Life Insurance Company, 1969.

APPENDIX IV

GENERAL REFERENCES

T HIS SUGGESTED LIST IS indicative of frequently used references in areas of interest to those concerned with nutrition. It is not intended to be inclusive in any category. The diet manuals listed are representative of the many fine manuals available. See lists at end of each section for references of primary interest in that section only.

Normal and Therapeutic Nutrition

Bauer, WW (Ed.): *Today's Health Guide. A Manual of Information and Guidance for the American Family,* revised. Chicago, Am Med Assoc, 1970.

Beeson, PB; McDermott, WJ (Eds.): *Cecil-Loeb Textbook of Medicine,* 13th ed. Philadelphia, Saunders, 1971. This book, written for physicians, includes detailed descriptions of diseases, laboratory diagnosis, and treatment.

Bland, JH: *Clinical Metabolism of Body Water and Electrolytes.* Philadelphia, Saunders, 1963.

Bogert, LJ; Briggs, GM; Calloway, DH: *Nutrition and Physical Fitness,* 9th ed. Philadelphia, Saunders, 1973. Emphasis is on the metabolic processes in normal nutrition.

Bondy, PK; Rosenberg, LE (Eds.): *Duncan's Diseases of Metabolism.* Philadelphia, Saunders, 1974. Provides descriptions of normal metabolism in man and alterations in disease.

Bourne, GE (Ed.): *World Review of Nutrition and Dietetics,* Vol. 13. New York, Karger, 1971.

Conn, H: *Current Therapy.* Philadelphia, Saunders, 1973. Concise information on current medical treatment with references to more detailed discussions. Section on nutrition.

Davidsohn, I; Henry, JB (Eds.): *Todd Sanford Diagnosis by Laboratory Methods,* 14th ed. Philadelphia, Saunders, 1969. Medical textbook describing diagnostic tests, normal values, and changes in disease.

Goodman, LS; Gilman, A (Eds.): *The Pharmacological Basis of Therapeutics,* 4th ed. New York, Macmillan, 1970. The mechanism of action of the nutrients furnished in foods, of drugs, and their interrelationships are detailed. References include many review articles as well as original reports on findings and newer concepts in treatment. Of particular interest to those concerned with clinical nutrition are the sections on water, salt, and ions; on drugs affecting renal function and electrolyte metabolism; and on vitamins.

Guthrie, HA: *Introductory Nutrition,* 2nd ed. St. Louis, Mosby, 1971. Normal nutrition with emphasis on understanding metabolic processes. Contains many tables, references, and a list of meanings of prefixes and suffixes used in nutrition.

Guyton, AC: *Textbook of Medical Physiology,* 4th ed. Philadelphia, Saunders, 1971. Sections on digestion, metabolism, and homeostatic mechanisms of the major functional systems are of particular interest to those concerned with nutrition.

Halpern, SL (Guest Ed.): Symposium on Current Concepts in Clinical Nutrition. *Med Clin North Am, 54:*1355, 1970. Entire issue (256 pages) devoted to current concepts on a broad range of subjects including trace elements, dental health, nutrition and aging, alcohol, and drug addiction. The section on nutrition and aging includes a discussion of the recommendations of the White House Conference.

Krause, MV; Hunscher, MA: *Food, Nutrition, and Diet Therapy,* 5th ed. Philadelphia, Saunders, 1972. In addition to information on foods and nutrition this textbook contains many tables, references, and other teaching aids.

Leverton, RM: *Food Becomes You.* Ames, Iowa, Iowa State Univ Press, 1965. Nutrition information presented in a practical and easy to read manner.

Mitchell, HS; Rynbergen, HJ; Anderson, L; Dibble, MV: *Cooper's Nutrition in Health and Disease,* 15th ed. Philadelphia, Lippincott, 1968. Contains many tables on food composition not readily found elsewhere, extensive references, and a glossary of terms to aid the beginning student.

National Academy of Sciences, National Research Council: *Recommended Dietary Allowances,* 8th ed. NAS-NRC. Washington, DC, 1974.

Pike, RS; Brown, MS: *Nutrition: An Integrated Approach.* New York, Wiley, 1967. Emphasis is on the intermediary metabolism to give the how and why of nutrition.

Robinson, C: *Normal and Therapeutic Nutrition,* 14th ed. New York, Macmillan, 1972. This book is a useful reference for many health professionals. Current nutrition practices and their biochemical bases are covered in this text. Easy-to-follow diet plans are included. Each chapter contains selected references and problems, and review questions useful in teaching. Included are new food composition tables of nutrients not listed in *USDA Handbook No 8,* lists of government publications, and other sources of teaching materials.

Robinson, JR: Water, the indispensible nutrient. *Nutr Today, 5* (no 1):16, 1970.

Stanbury, JB; Wyngaarden, JB; Fredrickson, DS (Eds.): *The Metabolic Basis of Inherited Disease,* 3rd ed. New York, McGraw Hill, 1972. Extensive and highly technical review of data by many research groups. Includes information on errors in metabolism that is difficult to find elsewhere. Many references.

Vivian, V: Nutrition Research Review. Series A, Edu-Pak 70. Chicago, *Am Diet Assoc,* 620 N Michigan Ave, Chicago, Illinois, 1971. This is a cassette-tape lecture.

White, A; Handler, P; Smith, EL: *Principles of Biochemistry,* 4th ed. New York, McGraw Hill, 1968. A graduate level textbook.

White House Conference on Food, Nutrition, and Health. Chairman, J Mayer. Washington, DC, Govt Printing Office, 1970. A report on the Dec 1969 conference with guidelines for action.

Williams, SR: *Nutrition and Diet Therapy.* St. Louis, Mosby, 1973. Contains many tables and references to the literature. Valuable information for the practicing dietitian.

Goodhart, RS; Shils, ME (Eds.): *Modern Nutrition in Health and Disease,* 5th ed. Philadelphia, Lea & Febiger, 1973. A basic reference book edited by physicians on the pathophysiology of disease. Each of the 40 chapters is written by a specialist in that area. Contains many tables, food plans, references to the literature, and other learning aids. For the physiological basis of diet therapy, this book is invaluable to the internist and the dietitian concerned with therapeutic nutrition.

Physical Disability

Klinger, JL; Frieden, FH; Sullivan, RA: *Mealtime Manual for the Aged and Handicapped.* New York, Essandess Special Editions, 1970. Compiled by the Institute of Rehabilitation Medicine, NYU Medical Center, as the result of a program funded by the Campbell Soup Fund to study the problems of the elderly and the handicapped in meal preparation and food service.

Diet Manuals and Tables of Food Composition

Adams, CF: *Nutritive Value of American Foods in Common Units.* USDA Agri Handbook No 456, In Press. Of particular value for weight-volume discussion.

Agri Research Service, USDA: *Nutritive Value of Foods,* revised. Home & Garden Bul 72, US Dept of Agriculture, Washington, DC, 1970. Composition of common foods in serving portions with weights of household measures in grams.

American Home Economics Association: *Handbook of Food Preparation,* 6th ed. Washington, DC, Am Home Econ Assoc, 1971. Contains information useful in calculating nutritive values of foods, particularly the weight, yield, and volume of market units of fresh and processed foods. Includes a table on the pH of common foods.

Am Hospital Assoc: *Food Service Manual for Health Care Institutions.*

Chicago, Am Hospital Assoc, 1972. Emphasis is on food service administration.

Browe, JH; Morley, DM; McCarthy, MC; Gofstein, RM: Diet and heart disease study in the cardiovascular health center. II: Construction of a food composition table and its use. *J Am Diet Assoc, 48*:101, 1966.

Church, CF; Church, HN: *Food Values of Portions Commonly Used,* 11th ed. Philadelphia, Lippincott, 1970. Nutrient content of many common and proprietary foods in terms of 26 nutrients and 8 essential amino acids. Data on brand-name products are included with the source of information; also sections on "vitamin-rich foods," dietary supplements, baby foods, combined foods, and alcoholic beverages.

Cincinnati Dietetic Association: *Cincinnati Diet Manual.* Cincinnati, 1968. Noteworthy for section on infant formulas and infant feeding.

Dawson, EH; Gilpin, GL; Fulton, LH: *Average Weight of a Measured Cup of Various Foods.* ARS 61-6 US Dept of Agriculture, Washington, DC, 1969. Weights of one cupful of drained solids and of solids and liquids of food products.

Depts of Dietetics: *Manual of Diets.* VA Hospital, West Haven, Connecticut; Yale-New Haven Hospital, New Haven, Connecticut, 1972. Manual from a large nutrition conscious medical center.

Galbraith, A; Hatch, L: *Diet Manual.* Boston, Massachusetts General Hospital, 1972. Manual from a large and renowned medical center.

McCance, RA; Widdowson, EM: *The Composition of Foods,* 3rd ed. Medical Research Council Spec Report Ser No 297. London, HM Stationery Office, 1960. This British publication includes several nutrients in addition to those found in most US food composition tables.

Manalo, R; Jones, JE: The content of constant diets. A comparison between analyzed and calculated values. *Am J Clin Nutr, 18*:339, 1966.

Mattice, MR: *Bridges' Food and Beverage Analyses,* 3rd ed. Philadelphia, Lea & Febiger, 1950. This general reference book, although not recent, contains much information hard to find elsewhere. Noteworthy are the sections on the pH of foods, and the data on copper, sulfur, iodine, chlorine, bromine, and purines.

Mayo Clinic Committee on Dietetics: *Mayo Clinic Diet Manual.* Philadelphia, Saunders, 1971. Comprehensive listing of therapeutic dietary programs at the Mayo Clinic. Includes some of the less frequently used diets and lists of foods in terms of special nutrients.

Ohlson, MA: *Experimental and Therapeutic Dietetics,* 2nd ed. Minneapolis, Burgess, 1972. Covers rationale, a discussion of nutrient content and patient acceptance as well as diet patterns. A widely used reference.

Page, L; Phipard, EF: *Essentials of an Adequate Diet.* HERR No 3, USDA, Washington, DC, 1957. Includes a short method of planning or checking for nutritional adequacy through selection of given amounts of foods of key nutritional value from each of the basic four food groups. Although the information is based on the 1953 Recommended Dietary Allowances, the method may be adapted to present use.

Peterkin, B; Evans, B: *Food Purchasing Guide.* Agri Handbook No 284, Agri Res Serv, USDA, Washington, DC, 1965. Information on weights of foods in market units, processing changes in weights, and yields in terms of servings per given portion weight.

Turner, D: *Handbook of Diet Therapy,* 5th ed. Chicago, Univ of Chicago Press, 1970. A reference manual of current dietetic principles compiled under the auspices of the American Dietetic Association. Food selection and diet plans to meet therapeutic needs are outlined, and references and food tables included.

Vanderbilt University Medical Center, Dept of Dietetics: *Diet Manual,* 2nd ed. Nashville, Vanderbilt Univ Press, 1969. Includes a wide range of diets and information on formulas and tube feedings.

Watt, BK; Merrill, AL: *Composition of Foods: Raw, Processed, Prepared,* revised. Agri Res Serv Handbook No 8, USDA, Washington, DC, 1963. Standard reference on American food composition in 100-gram and 1-pound units. This is a compilation of data from many research sources.

Food Preparation

National Institute of Health, Clinical Center: *A Dietetic Manual for Metabolic Kitchen Units.* HEW, Washington, DC, 1969.

Amino Acids

Block, RJ; Weiss, KW: *Amino Acid Handbook.* Springfield, Thomas, 1956.

Everson, GJ; Souders, HJ: Composition and nutritive importance of eggs. *J Am Diet Assoc, 33*:1244, 1957. (Includes amino acids, minerals, and vitamins of yolks and whites.)

FAO, United Nations: *Amino Acid Content of Foods and Biological Data on Proteins.* FAO Nutr Study No 24, Rome, 1970. (US distributor: Unipub, Inc, PO Box 433, New York, New York 10016.)

Harvey, DG: *Table of Amino Acids in Foods and Feeding Stuffs,* 2nd ed. Technical Communications no 19, Farnham Royal, England, Commonwealth Agricultural Bureaux, 1970.

McCarthy, MA; Orr, ML; Watt, BK: Phenylalanine and tyrosine in vegetables and fruits. *J Am Diet Assoc, 52*:130, 1968.

Miller, GT; Williams, VR; Moschette, DS: Phenylalanine content of fruit. *J Am Diet Assoc, 46*:43, 1965.

Munro, HN (Ed.): *Mammalian Protein Metabolism,* Vol IV. New York, Academic Press, 1970.

Orr, ML; Watt, BK: *Amino Acid Content of Foods.* HERR No 4, Agri Res Serv, USDA, Washington, DC, 1957.

Fats

Bickel, JH; Gray, JC: *A Low Cholesterol Diet Manual.* Iowa City, Univ of Iowa, 1968.

Feeley, RM; Criner, PE; Watt, BK: Cholesterol content of foods. *J Am Diet Assoc, 61*:134, 1972.

Goddard, VR; Goodall, L: *Fatty Acids in Food Fats.* HERR No 7, Agri Res Serv, USDA, Washington, DC, 1959.

Hardinge, MG; Crooks, H: Fatty acid composition of food fats. *J Am Diet Assoc, 34*:1065, 1958.

Carbohydrates

Hardinge, MG; Swarner, JB; Crooks, H: Carbohydrates in foods. *J Am Diet Assoc, 46*:197, 1965.

Minerals

Comar, CL; Bronner, F: *Mineral Metabolism: An Advanced Treatise.* III Supplementary volume. New York, Academic Press, 1969.

Davies, IJT: *Clinical Significance of Essential Biologic Metals.* London, Heinemann Medical Books, 1972.

Gormican, A: Inorganic elements in foods used in hospital menus. *J Am Diet Assoc, 56*:397, 1970.

Mertz, W; Cornatzer, WE (Eds.): *Newer Trace Elements in Nutrition.* New York, Mercel Dekker, Inc, 1971.

Prasad, AS; Oberleas, D; Rajasakaran, G: Essential micronutrient elements. *Am J Clin Nutr, 23*:581, 1970.

Raisz, LG: Calcium metabolism—recent advances. DM: *Disease-a-Month,* Dec 1972.

Sandstead, HH, et al: Current concepts on trace minerals. *Med Clin North Am, 54*:1509, 1970.

Underwood, EJ: *Trace Elements in Animal and Human Nutrition,* 3rd ed. New York, Academic Press, 1971.

Zook, EG: Mineral composition of fruits. I: Edible yield, total solids and ash of 30 fresh fruits. *J Am Diet Assoc, 52*:218, 1968.

————: Mineral composition of fruits. III: Total solids, ash, nitrogen, and minerals of six dried fruits. *J Am Diet Assoc, 53*:588, 1968.

————; Lehman, J: Mineral composition of fruits. II: Nitrogen, calcium, phosphorus, potassium, aluminum, boron, copper, iron, manganese, sodium. *J Am Diet Assoc, 52*:225, 1968.

Chromium

Mertz, W: Chromium occurrence and function in biological systems. *Physiol Rev, 49*:163, 1969.

Cobalt

Schroeder, HA, et al: Essential trace elements in man: Cobalt. *J Chronic Dis, 20*:869, 1967.

Copper

Hook, L; Brandt, IK: Copper content of some low copper foods. *J Am Diet Assoc, 49*:202, 1966.

Pennington, JT; Calloway, DH: Copper content of foods. *J Am Diet Assoc, 63*:143, 1973.

Schroeder, HA, et al: Essential trace elements in man: Copper. *J Chronic Dis, 19*:1007, 1966.

Magnesium

Hathaway, ML: *Magnesium in Human Nutrition.* HERR No 19, Agri Res Serv, USDA, Washington, DC, 1962.

Nelson, GY; Gram, MR: Magnesium content of accessory foods. *J Am Diet Assoc, 38*:437, 1961.

Schroeder, HA; Nason, AP; Tipton, IH: Essential metals in man: Magnesium. *J Chronic Dis, 21*:815, 1969.

Wacker, WE: Magnesium metabolism. *N Engl J Med, 278*:712, 1968.

Manganese

Schroeder, HA; Balassa, JJ; Tipton, IH: Essential trace elements in man: Manganese. A study in homeostasis. *J Chronic Dis, 19*:545, 1966.

Potassium

Snively, WD; Westerman, RL: The clinician views potassium deficit. *Minn Med, 48*:713, 1965.

Selenium

Morris, VC; Levander, OA: Selenium content of food. *J Nutr, 100*:1383, 1970.

Vitamins

DeLuca, HF; Suttie, JW (Eds.): *The Fat Soluble Vitamins.* Madison, Wis, Univ of Wis Press, 1969.

Food and Agriculture Organization: *Requirement for Vitamin A, Thiamine, Riboflavin and Niacin.* FAO Nutr Meetings Rept Series No 41, WHO Tech Rept Series No 326, 1967.

Sebrell, WH; Harris RS (Eds.): *The Vitamins,* Vol 5, 2nd ed. New York, Academic Press, 1972.

Stein, M: *Vitamins.* Baltimore, Williams and Wilkins, 1971.

Note: Although addressed to problems encountered in parenteral nutrition, the American Medical Association *Symposium on Total Parenteral Nutrition* (1972) is a compendium of information on the present (1973) state of knowledge concerning the nutritional requirements of man. Each section includes references.

Commercial Sources of Dietary Foods and Technical Information on Special Ingredients

Anderson, TA; Fomon, SJ: Commercially prepared strained and junior foods for infants. *J Am Diet Assoc, 58*:520, 1971.

Chicago Dietetic Supply House, Inc, 405 E Shawmut Ave, La Grange, Ill 60525. Variety of foods for modified diets including wheat starch and low protein, low electrolyte products.

Doyle Pharmaceutical Co, Hwy 100 at W 23 St, Minneapolis, Minn 55416.
Resource Low Protein Baking Mix, Controlyte protein-free caloric
supplement, tube feeding.

Eaton Laboratories, Norwich, New York. Vivonex.

General Mills, Inc, Chemical Division, 4620 W 77 St, Minneapolis, Minn
55435. Paygel-P® wheat starch and other products for modified diets.

Gerber Products Co, Fremont, Michigan 49412. Tube feedings, foods for
infants, children; foods for modified diets.

Institutional and Industrial Kosher Products Directory, 3rd ed. (1972)
Union of Orthodox Jewish Congregations of America, 84 Fifth Ave,
New York City 10011. Listing of over 2000 Rabinically endorsed and
supervised kosher products.

Loma Linda Foods, Mount Vernon, Ohio 43050. Low phenylalanine foods.

Mead Johnson Laboratories, Evansville, Indiana 47721. Lofenalac®, a low
phenylalanine food; Portagen, medium chain triglycerides; Prosobee,
soy isolate milk.

Riker Laboratories, Northridge, California 91325. Edial, medium chain
triglycerides.

This is not intended to be a complete list. There are many others;
consult current journals. Some companies have also prepared exchange values for their products.

DIET IN HEALTH AND DISEASE

Addendum

Ileal resection to decrease caloric absorption in morbid obesity has created life threatening hazards in some persons. The ileum is a major site of nutrient absorption.

Fromm (1973) discussed the pathophysiology and treatment. He listed the major effects of ileal resection as steatorrhea, diarrhea, an increased incidence of cholelithiasis and renal calculi, and vitamin B_{12} deficiency.

The ileum is the main area of bile acid absorption. Fecal losses govern the rate of liver bile acid synthesis. When bile acids are not absorbed they appear in the feces increasing the rate of liver synthesis. With extensive ileal resection resulting in high fecal losses of bile acids, hepatic synthesis cannot keep pace with the losses, resulting in a diminished bile acid pool. Steatorrhea follows. With an increased amount of bile acids entering the colon, electrolyte and water secretion is stimulated with a diarrhea following.

Cholestyramine, an anion exchange resin, will decrease the diarrhea by sequestering the acids. This process prevents their reabsorption further depleting the available bile salts. Patients with longer ileal resection respond less well to cholestyramine. This appears to be due to the severe steatorrhea with an increased amount of long chain fatty acids passing into the colon. These fatty acids inhibit water absorption and may be hydroxalated by bacterial enzymes to cause diarrhea.

Substitution of medium chain triglycerides for the long chain triglycerides will decrease the steatorrhea with extensive, or less extensive ileal resection. The patient with *less* extensive resection will continue to have diarrhea, Dr. Fromm says, regardless of the form of the fat, because the unabsorbed bile acid, rather than the fat is the major cause of the diarrhea.

A decrease in bile acids to solubilize cholesterol causes an in-

277

crease in gallstones. It also is associated with an increased incidence of renal calculi. Renal stones contain oxalate which is thought to be derived from bile acids by the action of bacterial enzymes and conversion to oxalic acid in the liver.

Stauffer et al (1973) suggest that the hyperoxaluria is related to enhanced absorption of dietary oxalate. They reported a dramatic decrease in oxalate excretion with the use of a diet containing less than 10 mg per day of oxalate. The diet consisted of Flexical and roast beef or chicken. They also found the elemental diet effective.

Zarembski and Hodgkinson (1962) reported the oxalic acid content of English diets.

Vitamin B_{12} malabsorption is related to the extent and site of the ileal resection. The 15 inches of ileum just proximal to the ileocecal valve is the most active site of vitamin B_{12} absorption.

Treatment of symptoms noted is primarily medical. Diet is palliative at best. If symptoms are severe, an elemental (chemically defined) diet is warranted. A high carbohydrate, high protein, low fat diet is indicated. If laboratory tests show hyperoxaluria, limit the oxalic acid content as much as is consistent with nutritional goals. If symptoms do not respond to medication, lean meat plus an elemental diet may be the answer. Multiple vitamin and mineral therapy (included in the elemental diet) is necessary.

REFERENCES

Fromm, D.: Ileal resection, or disease, and the blind loop syndrome: Current concepts of pathophysiology. *Surgery, 73*:639, 1973.

Stauffer, JQ, et al: Acquired hyperoxaluria with regional enteritis after ileal resection. *Ann Int Med, 79*:383, 1973.

Zarembski, PM; Hodgkinson, A: The oxalic acid content of English diets. *Br J Nutr, 16*:627, 1962.

INDEX

279

food for infants, 41
food for toddlers, 44
Frederickson
  (see Hyperlipoproteinemia)
galactosemia, 192
hyperlipoproteinemia, 175
ketogenic, 199
lactation, 37
lactose restricted, 189, 190
liquid, clear, full, 53, 55
pregnancy, 34
protein modifications
  gluten restricted, 150
  high protein, 101
  low protein, 102
  low protein-low potassium, 112
  phenylalanine restricted, 141
residue, low, 78
smooth, 78
sodium controlled, 206, 207
soft, and modifications, 78
surgery
  following cardiac surgery, 41
  following gastric surgery (for
    dumping syndrome), 82
  following peridontal surgery, 66
  preceding surgery, 66
  tube feedings, 57
Diets in diagnostic procedures
  allergy elimination diet, 220
  calcium, 200 mg constant, 222
  cholecystogram, fat-free supper, 224
  fat absorption, 223
  glucose tolerance, 225
  non-protein breakfast for
    Schilling test, 226
  tryptophan metabolic studies, 226
Diverticulosis, 66
Drugs and body processes
  B₆ and L-dopa, 243
  electrolyte loss in diuretic therapy, 133
  monoamine oxidase inhibitors, 242
Dumping syndrome, 82

E

Elemental diet, 59
Equivalent weight of electrolytes, 265
Exchanges
  cholesterol, 164
  food exchange system, 14
    bread, 18
    fats, 22
    fruits, 17
    meat, poultry, fish, eggs, 20
    milk, 15
    vegetables, 16
    meat, lean, 22
    phenylalanine, 143
    protein-electrolyte, 116

F

Fat(s)
  cholesterol, 164
  consumption in U.S., 182, 183
  diets low in (*see* Calories)
  exchanges, 22
  "modified fat" meaning, 171
  percentage contribution in
    hospital diets, 182
  polyunsaturated
    in vegetable oils, 251
    vitamin E in fat, 251
  saturated, 161
Fiber, 77
Fluid(s)
  adult requirement, 14
  infant formulas, 41
  intake, calculation, control
    during oliguria, 106-109
Folacin (folic acid,
    pteroylglutamic acid), 257
Food exchange system, 14
  (*see* Exchanges)
Formulas, infant, 39

G

Galactose, galactosemia, 192
Glucose tolerance test, 225
Gluten, 150
Gout (*see* Low purine diet)

H

Height-weight tables for
  men and women, 267
Hyperkinesis, 242
Hyperlipoproteinemia, 175
Hyperoxaluria, 277

I

Ileal bypass, 277
Infant feeding
  dietary allowances, 4, 5
  foods added at various ages, 41
  formula calculations, 39
  use of iron-fortified foods, 40
Iodine, 14
Iron
  increased need during pregnancy, 35